00 may 11

D0426859

TALK SOFTLY

A Memoir

TALK SOFTLY

A Memoir

CYNTHIA O'NEAL

Seven Stories Press

NEW YORK

Seven Stories Press
140 Watts Street
New York, NY 10013
www.sevenstories.com

In Canada: Publishers Group Canada, 559 College Street, Suite 402, Toronto, ON M6G 1A9

In the UK: Turnaround Publisher Services Ltd., Unit 3, Olympia Trading Estate, Coburg Road, Wood Green, London N22 6TZ

In Australia: Palgrave Macmillan, 15–19 Claremont Street, South Yarra, VIC 3141

College professors may order examination copies of Seven Stories Press titles for a free six-month trial period. To order, visit http://www.sevenstories.com/textbook or send a fax on school letterhead to (212) 226-1411.

Book design by Jon Gilbert

Library of Congress Cataloging-in-Publication Data

O'Neal, Cynthia, 1934-
  Talk softly : a memoir / Cynthia O'Neal. -- Seven Stories Press 1st ed.
    p. cm.
  ISBN 978-1-58322-906-4 (hardcover)
  1. O'Neal, Cynthia, 1934- 2. O'Neal, Cynthia, 1934---Marriage. 3. O'Neal, Cynthia, 1934---Friends and associates. 4. AIDS (Disease)--Patients--Counseling of--New York (State)--New York. 5. Counselors--New York (State)--New York--Biography. 6. Friends in Deed (Organization) 7. Care of the sick--Case studies. 8. Life change events--United States--Case studies. 9. Loss (Psychology)--Case studies. 10. Husbands--Death--Psychological aspects--Case studies. I. Title.
  RC606.55.054A3 2010
  362.196'97920092--dc22
  [B]   2009047606

Printed in the United States of America

9 8 7 6 5 4 3 2 1

For Patrick
For Max and Fitz

I see now that all of it matters. Everything counts.

CHAPTER 1

While I do not keep a diary or journal of any kind, in my early twenties I did begin saving my appointment books. Recently, out of a specific curiosity, I opened the one for 1971. It fell open to a week in May that recorded a life that now seems so distant, so other, that I barely recognize it.

As I read the daily entries, while there were many things I wasn't able to remember—what was the name of the film that Patrick and I saw that Saturday night?—I did remember how very important every bit of it seemed at the time.

We were living in a brownstone on West Seventy-first Street in New York City—the "we" being my husband, Patrick O'Neal, our two sons, Max and Fitz, and me. We'd been in that house for almost ten years and were soon to leave it for the simple reason that I had burned out on stairs. Our sons had exquisite timing: precisely as my foot hit the first floor I'd hear a voice from the third floor—*"Mom!"* I wanted to live horizontally instead of vertically, and fortunately Patrick agreed.

One entry that week recorded a meeting we were having with a building contractor; the meeting was to take place in the apartment we had just bought but not yet moved into, and for which we had

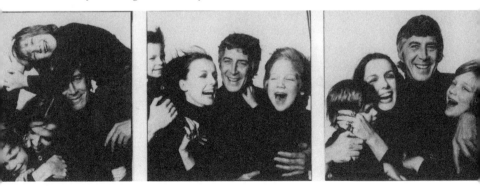

extensive renovation plans. The apartment was in the Dakota, and we were excited about the move. To me the Dakota was the most desirable place to live in all of New York City, and given my passion for New York City, that would translate into the most desirable place in all the world. Not only do the big apartments have high ceilings, rich moldings, glowing wood paneling, marble fireplaces—the works—we would also have all those glamorous neighbors: Lauren Bacall, Felicia and Leonard Bernstein, John Lennon. I remember it seemed to me that by actually living in the building where John Lennon lived some great thing had been achieved.

I see that on the Wednesday there was a parent-teacher meeting at Bank Street School—the end-of-the-school-year wrap-up. I'd written down the time of the appointment and then "Fitz" in parentheses. I'd also written the word "bread." Obviously that was the year Fitz's teacher showed us a little booklet he'd made. The students were told to make a six-page booklet, one page for each year of their lives. They then had to illustrate what they thought was the most important event of that year (they could consult with their parents on the first couple of years). For year four Fitz had drawn a loaf of brown bread and written, "This was the year my mother started giving us brown bread." For year five he drew the same loaf of bread and wrote, "This is the year I started to like brown bread."

There was a dentist appointment and one with my dressmaker, Mary Fukui. I also saw that we'd had dinner with Phyllis and Adolph Green on Tuesday at The Ginger Man, the restaurant we owned with Patrick's brother, Mike, and his wife Chris. Patrick and I saw *A Touch of the Poet* on Wednesday night, watched a softball game in Central Park with our boys on Saturday afternoon, and went to a movie by ourselves later that evening.

Then there was the big event of the week, written in large block letters: RUDOLF—DINNER HERE, which meant that that Friday night we were having a small dinner party for Rudolf Nureyev after his performance with the Royal Ballet at the Met. It also meant that while I didn't write down any particular notes about it, I'm sure I spent a good part of that week focused on that dinner—figuring out a meal that I could mostly prepare before we went to the ballet and finish when we got home—intent on it being the most perfect evening possible. For me, that would include making the whole thing look completely effortless. Seeing Nureyev, on- and offstage, was one of the great excitements of life in those days—and nothing to do with Rudolf was even remotely effortless. He was consistently and lavishly entertained all over the world by the very rich and famous, in homes where everything was impeccably done by a well-trained staff. In our home, the staff was me.

Rudolf always had to have a perfect blood-rare steak at the ready for his dinner—some idea about the red meat giving him strength and energy. So I'd prepare whatever it was I was making for everyone else, be ready to throw his steak on the fire when the moment came, and then Rudolf would look at the dinner the rest of us were having and decide that that's what he wanted after all, and the dog would end up with the steak. That's how it happened every single time, but I never had the nerve to not have the steak.

Another night, when Max was about five, Rudolf walked in with a great-looking young guy and a large heavy burlap sack that a fan had given him. The great-looking guy he introduced as Wallace Bean Potts ("Bean" to us forever more). Then he walked to the middle of the living room, opened the sack, and out came three enormous lobsters, which began crawling around the floor. Hearing the commotion, our son Max came flying down the stairs, glanced at the lobsters with a total lack of surprise, and said, "Hello, Rudolf! You still dancing?" The look on Rudolf's face! He was furious! Even a five-year-old child should have known that the great Rudolf Nureyev was still dancing!

That's what my life looked like.

MAY 1971

CHAPTER 2

From where I'm standing off to the side of the room, I can watch the people as they file in and take their seats. Several dozen young men in their twenties or thirties, a few older men, and three or four women. The seriousness of what brings these people together is apparent—it's heavy in the air.

There are those who arrive alone and those who enter in small groups of two or three, talking to each other as they scan the room, deciding where they want to sit. Some appear sure of themselves, full of purpose, and some are visibly tentative, not at all convinced they want to be here.

The men and women who to all outward appearances are doing well are not the ones I'm focused on at this moment. I have my eye out for the visibly unsure, the discernibly fragile.

I watch one man come in by himself who looks to be a little older than most of the other people in this room—probably close to fifty. The room is filling rapidly, and I wonder how he is going to find a place to sit as he seems unable to take his eyes off the floor.

Right behind him is a very young, extremely handsome man who holds his head high and walks with his hand resting on the shoulder of the man in front of him. He is being guided because obviously his sight is going or gone. He will not be the only person here tonight of whom that is true.

I spot one extremely thin pale kid in a sweat suit, walking with a cane and moving very slowly as though every atom of his body were in pain. My guess is that that soft sweat suit is all he can bear to hang on his wire coat hanger of a body.

Every possible visual style is represented in this room, from conservative-looking businessmen in their Paul Stuart suits who look as if they have just gotten off the subway up from Wall Street—and some have done exactly that—to one blond man with hair halfway down his back, plucked eyebrows, multiple pierced earrings, and a ring on every finger.

There's a very sad-looking little man wearing plaid trousers and a frayed Windbreaker sitting right next to a real knockout with jet black hair, clothing to match, and a brilliant red scarf knotted around his neck. There are tweed jackets, tattoos, shaved heads, nylon sports gear, cashmere turtlenecks, and black leather. There are also a lot of men who look like they could be the guy standing next to you at the deli.

I watch several people who have been to these groups before head immediately for the seat they always take; they have staked out their piece of geography—third row, fourth seat from the end, seventh row on the aisle . . . The ones who look really uncomfortable usually try to grab a chair in the very last row in hopes that they won't be noticed. Over the months, I have grown used to certain faces in certain places.

I like to stand off to the side and simply witness this part of the evening. If I stay in my office until it's time to lead the group, I will miss a lot of information. These are unguarded moments—the set of the face, the way people hold their bodies and move, their animation or lack of it as they speak to a friend—these can tell me things they may not choose to talk about later during the group. By just quietly observing I can form my own list of those I hope will raise their hands, and if they don't, I may try to have a private word with them after the group.

Without knowing for sure, without going around the room and asking the question, it's a pretty safe bet that the great majority of these young men and women are infected with the AIDS virus or, in some cases, that they are the friends, lovers, spouses, or partners of someone who is infected with the AIDS virus.

Some of the people in this room look perfectly healthy, some look ill—some look very ill. There are those who are alarmingly thin as a product of wasting syndrome—that aspect of the AIDS infection where the pounds just keep melting away no matter how much food is forced down, a few whose faces are marked with the dark oblongs of Kaposi's sarcoma—the kind of skin cancer that can take hold when the immune system is too weak to combat it. There are those who are bald under their knitted woolen caps as a result of chemotherapy, and three or four who have the look in their eyes of someone who will soon be leaving this life. It's a look I have come to recognize. There are men I have never seen before and men I have also seen in their homes, in their hospital beds, or in the surreal surroundings of the ICU. Still, my relationship with most of them has been contained within the walls of this room.

Back in the spring of 1987, I began meeting and getting to know hundreds of people who were HIV positive. I found their circumstance—being very young and being told they would most likely die soon—extremely affecting. I was impressed by their courage and moved by their compassion—the beautiful way in which they took care of one another. To one degree or another I cared about every single one of them, and I most certainly care about every client here at Friends In Deed. I've not yet found a way to like all of them—sometimes there is a personality or an attitude that is so tough for me to deal with I'd like to run right out of the room, but then, as I get to know them, as I see the fear behind the behavior, I do eventually arrive at love. I often wish I could get there more quickly.

The meeting, which I will be facilitating, is to start at 7:00, and just a couple of minutes before the hour, I see my husband, Patrick, walk through the door. This organization, Friends In Deed, has been open for about five months, and a few days ago I mentioned to Patrick that I thought I was ready for him to come and sit in on one of the Tuesday-night Big Groups. He's never before seen me lead a group. For that matter, he's not been with me in the hospital room of a young man dying of AIDS, he's not accompanied me on a home visit to a very ill client, nor has he ever heard me speak at a memorial service. My husband does not participate actively in this life I've chosen, but he absolutely supports it. He does not complain when we don't have dinner until very late at night, he steps up and does more with our boys when I'm not around, and he's understanding when I'm a mess because someone I have grown very fond of dies. More I could not ask.

I watch him take a seat way in the back corner, guessing correctly that I am nervous about his being here. I very much care what he will think. I would like him to be proud of me.

It's time to begin. I move to the center of the room and look over the faces in front of me. For one moment my breath catches—when I glance at Patrick I see that he looks just as ill as many of the other people in the room—he's lost weight, he's pale, and something has happened around the eyes. He is not HIV positive, however he does have Epstein-Barr syndrome, which is also an autoimmune disease, one that leaves him weak and tired to the point of exhaustion most of the time. The symptoms have certainly affected his life and therefore mine, but we have not related to it as something to be really frightened about, simply as something to cure. When I look at him now, I know in my heart that something is very wrong. Of necessity, I push that knowledge away and go to work.

When everyone notices that I have moved to the front of the room, the talking winds down and there is a short silence. I welcome the group to Friends In Deed, lead them into a short meditation designed to quiet and center, remind them of our commitment to respect the anonymity of everyone in the room, and follow that with a few necessary announcements and a brief explanation of our agenda for the evening. Then the first clients begin to raise their hands. They tell us what's going on in their lives, what they're having a particularly tough time with at the moment, I respond, there is a dialogue between the two of us, and then we move on to the next person. At first, I'm very aware of Patrick, but soon the work itself takes over and I almost forget he's here.

Mike is the first to raise his hand, as he almost always is. He's from a family of five sons. Two have already died of AIDS and Mike, too, has the virus. Sean tells us that he has a new health crisis, which he does not specifically name, and my heart sinks. He has already had a liver transplant as well as several other surgeries and procedures. I wonder how much more his body can tolerate. Rebecca tells us how ill she is from the side effects of the medications she's been given. Richard talks about what's happening to him, the slow deterioration of his physical body and also what he feels is happening to his mind as a result of his AIDS-related toxoplasmosis; he says that he doesn't think he can tolerate losing everything that defines him as a human being, and he may well opt to end his life before that happens. Carlos talks about the fact that his mother is coming to New York and he can't sleep with worrying about whether or not to reveal his HIV status to her, something he has avoided thus far; he predicts that the news will destroy his mother's life, that she does not have the emotional strength to handle the truth, yet he is very uncomfortable with keeping such a secret from his mother whom he loves very much. Jack tells us that he's been having unsafe sex and he knows he should get tested but he's too frightened to do so. Barry tells us that his partner died ten months ago and that he himself is absolutely paralyzed with grief; he thinks he should be better by now but he simply cannot get over the loss. Jamal says that he came to New York a few years ago, formed a group of nine close friends, and now every single one of them is dead; he is the sole survivor and he cannot conceive of making new intimate friends at this point in his life; his loneliness and isolation are unbearable. Gordon says the pain from his neuropathy is excruciating twenty-four hours a day and the pain meds don't even touch it.

I do not tell anyone what to do. That is not my job—it is not what we do here at Friends In Deed. My job is to support the clients in trusting their own instincts and strengths, to remind them that we all have a place deep within us that knows what is right for us, that they can gather information and listen to opinions but the bottom line is they are the ones responsible for their own bodies and lives. I remind them that we are gathered together in the Big Groups to support and empower one another in using whatever it is that we are given to deal with as a vehicle to transform our lives—to make us more conscious and compassionate human beings. I assure them that there is no "right" way to grieve—that grief is entirely individual. We discuss the fact that if they look they will see that their fears are always about the future, what they are telling themselves *could* happen. When I ask them how they are right this very minute, the answer is almost always the same: *Well, sitting here right now I'm okay, but* . . . We look at how easy it is to destroy any possibility of serenity or joy in this day by living in negative predictions regarding a day that isn't even here yet, and in truth we never really know what will happen until it happens. I also remind them that their physical body is not who they are and their disease is not who they are—*who* they are is a beautiful magnificent spirit. There are many other things as well, but these are some of the principles that seem to come up at every meeting.

It's been a very intense hour and a half. To lighten things up a bit before we close, I quote a line from my one of my teachers, Ram Dass, and remind them that their physical body is only the Ford they've been driving around town in.

The meeting is a typical Friends In Deed Big Group.

When the meeting ends I look around for Patrick and he, cool dude that he always is, does not rush over—rather, we make our way slowly through the crowd, stopping and talking to people as we go. When we are finally standing, looking at each other, he says . . .

"When did this happen?"

It was a good question. All the next day I thought about it and the seriousness of the look on my husband's face when he asked me the question. I think about it still. Patrick had watched me become more and more involved with the AIDS community over the preceding years, and I imagine that he'd most likely been picturing me in the role of administrator/organizer. I suppose that watching me actually standing there at the head of a large packed room, facilitating a group of nearly a hundred people, dealing with life-and-death issues, put the whole thing in a new light. Perhaps he saw that I had acquired certain skills he didn't know I had. Also, why wouldn't he be confused by how much my focus in life had changed? In the thirty-five years we'd been together, when had I ever demonstrated any leaning toward helping other people, when had he ever seen me perform even a single act of service outside my own family and our very closest friends? The answer is simple—he hadn't. And now, there I was—a kind of noncredentialed professional.

I suspect our friends shared some of Patrick's puzzlement. There are many good longtime friends who had known me as someone who was most often focused on such important matters as finding the perfect Italian shoes, the perfect frame for the picture, the perfect black satin jacket, the perfect wine for the coq au vin, the best possible seats for opening night—what must any of them have thought when I canceled our dinner date because instead I was choosing to spend my evening in the emergency room with someone I barely knew?

Still thinking about Patrick's reaction and before going to work the next morning, I visited an AIDS patient, Ernesto, in the hospital— something I have done times without number over the years. When I go into a hospital I can never be sure what I will find. I have left people of an evening sitting up having their dinner, talking about going home, and come back the next day to find them delirious with fever and moaning with pain. I've also said good night to people who couldn't lift their heads from the pillow and found them doing the *New York Times* crossword puzzle the next morning. As with everything else, I am sure of nothing.

That morning I walked through the automatic doors. I recognized the faces behind the reception desk, and they recognized me. I gave them Ernesto's name and room number, they didn't bother to check—they knew I knew. Spellman, seventh floor, AIDS unit. I walked down corridors I had walked down hundreds of times. I knew every inch of them. I knew the smell. I knew every elevator, which ones worked better than others, and when to take the stairs. I got to room 707, and not for the first time. Tomato Bob had been in that very room. And Pam. And Ian. And Richard, And Steven. And Mark. And Brazilian John. I walked in with soft steps and looked at Ernesto in the bed. He was asleep with his left hand on the control button of a pump that would shoot a dose of Dilaudid into his veins. For pain. At that point he was hitting the button about every eight minutes. I put my hand over his heart. He opened his eyes and put his arms out to me. After we hugged he told me what was happening. The doctors thought that the terrible pain in his chest and left shoulder could be cancer again; they didn't know if it was a recurrence of the old cancer or a new cancer—or maybe, please god, it was only PCP pneumonia. When they did know, they would begin to treat it. Ernesto told me that he was fine—he told me that he was not dying. I believed him. I also believed that if and when he was dying, he would know that too—and he would still be fine.

Ernesto could have been the Friends In Deed poster boy. He had been coming to our Big Groups every week; he asked for one-on-one counseling when he felt he needed it. He believed that whatever happened was meant to happen; he knew in the deepest part of him that he was much more than his physical body. He was calm and centered and present. He worked hard to find as much delight in each day as he possibly could. He inspired us all.

We talked awhile. I looked hard into his beautiful golden Venezuelan face with the almost-black Picasso eyes. He was tired and medication fuzzy, so I didn't stay long. As I walked down the halls, rode the elevator, and headed for the exit, all the hundreds of

Saint Vincent's hours that I had spent rode with me. I felt them in my shoulders and in the back of my neck and in my belly. When I stepped outside onto the New York City street, I paused for a few seconds, almost confused, as though I suddenly found myself in a city I'd never seen before.

As it happens, after visiting a client at Saint Vincent's and then heading east toward Friends In Deed, I pass our very first apartment, the one we moved into in 1958; it's right there on West Twelfth Street, just a few strides from the door to the hospital.

I have often done what I did that morning—stood there and looked up at the windows of what was once our apartment on the parlor floor. Sometimes I just glance at the windows to see if the drapes we hung all those years ago are still there. Miraculously they were—they still are. They are the color of butter and they were made for us by a tiny little bird of a woman with a great thin beak of a nose, named Lotte Sunshine, who would immediately look at anything I'd bought and say, "Whadcha pay?" Then, with the slightest twitch of her eyebrows, Lotte would make it clear that I was a fool and I'd paid too much. Looking at those drapes, it occurred to me that if I walked through the door maybe all the rest would be there too—the black marble fireplaces, the high ceilings with their heavy moldings, our first pieces of antique furniture, the big shaggy white dog. Maybe Patrick and I would be there.

I focused on the stairs leading up to the front door; I imagined being twenty-two years old again running up and down those stairs— running to a photographer's studio for that day's booking, running to the market, running to meet Patrick at the movies.

I tried to remember the life that went on in those rooms. Images floated to the surface in quick succession. The first image was of Patrick and me sitting at our round table having dinner with a couple of friends when suddenly there was a great clap of thunder in the night sky and our dog, who'd been lying peacefully nearby, took one great terrified arcing leap that landed him right in the middle of the table. We now had an enormous white standard poodle standing with his paws planted among the plates and glasses.

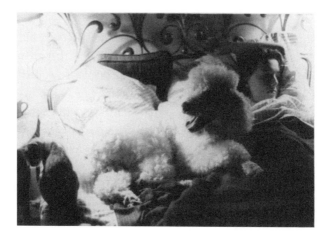

I remembered a party we gave for some members of the Actors Studio to which Norman Mailer came and brought along a scruffy-looking young man who went around the apartment taking the cigarettes out of the cigarette boxes and putting them in his pockets. It was a sour note in the lovely party for which I'd worked so hard, and also the young man had a generally loose-cannon feel about him, so I finally said something to Norman, who slowly traced his fingers across my forehead and said, "You have a fine noble brow, and you shouldn't concern yourself with such things." There was one night when Patrick and I had a fierce argument and I stormed out of the apartment, slamming doors as I went. Then, after walking the neighborhood for a while, I crept back into the apartment, quietly lay down on our sofa, barely breathing, intent on Patrick not hearing me so that he would be frantic with worry. I needn't have bothered—I could hear him softly snoring. I could remember being in our bedroom the night before John F. Kennedy's inauguration and being so excited I couldn't sleep because we were going to Washington, to be there, to be witness. I said to Patrick, "This is terrible—we'll be exhausted—why can't I sleep?" "It's okay," he said, "you're just journey proud." "Journey proud"—what does that mean? Just what's happening right now, the great excitement before a journey.

Standing there all those many years later, I wondered what I was like when I lived there? Hard to imagine. I remembered that I was hungry for an interesting, exciting life, the kind of life my mother often spoke of with sadness and longing—the kind of life she did not have and that I do have. I thought about my mother a lot in those days and how excited she would have been by my New York life—how she could have bragged to her friends!

Whatever dreams I dreamed on the other side of those windows I was looking at—my intense desire to be right in the middle of all that New York City is—whatever those dreams were, there was one thing I was sure of: they did not include anything like the AIDS epidemic.

When I got home from work at the end of that day, it wasn't all that late but Patrick was already asleep. He slept a lot in those days. Maybe he'd wake up in a while and if he did, I'd cook some dinner, but meanwhile, because I couldn't get his question out of my mind, I pulled out a videotape, a copy of an ancient home movie my brother had sent me some months before, and snapped it into the VCR. I sat down to watch, to search for clues, to look for some answers.

HOME MOVIE

The figures on the screen moved with a twitching stop-start motion. I watched a very little boy toddle along the sidewalk then sit down hard on his padded bottom. Get up. Three more steps—down. Now he was in a playpen, set outdoors, in the middle of a lawn.

An older but still very young girl with two enormous hair bows on top of her head, sat next to the playpen—alternately reaching in and making some gesture toward the boy, taking his hand for an instant, then turning and smiling self-consciously at the camera.

Next the girl was walking along the sidewalk holding the hand of a man wearing a double-breasted suit and a fedora. They walked toward the camera, then away from it, looking back over their shoulders, smiling and talking. We don't hear what they're saying.

A woman walked out of a house and down the front path, chin held high, smiling—a star making her entrance.

Now a quick cut, and suddenly we were on a beach. The same woman walked from the edge of the ocean up onto the sand toward a towel spread a few feet from the farthest reach of the waves. She was wearing a yellow one-piece bathing suit, walking way up on the tips of her toes. When she sat down on the towel, she lost her balance, rocked backward, legs flying in the air.

Another quick cut to a rowboat on a lake surrounded by mountains. The girl had a very small fish on the end of a line and more great big hair bows, as if two enormous butterflies had landed on her head.

The rest of the film cut back and forth between the house and yard seen in the beginning, and the mountain-encircled lake and woods. There were times when, strangely, the background was clear and bright, and the figures in the foreground were so heavily shadowed it was difficult to make them out. Other times the whole scene was almost completely white as if all color had been leached by a fierce burning sun. So it alternated between the people appearing to be in hiding, shadowed, and up to no good—then, with their jerky motions, looking anguished in some terrible flesh-melting heat. This home movie had been made a long time ago. It was very low-tech.

This was my family. I was the one with the bows in my hair. The man was my father, Robert Earl Baxter (always called "Pawnee" by me and my brother because I once found a school report he'd written and signed "Pawnee Bob"), the woman, my mother, Helen

Komaromy Baxter, and the little boy was my younger brother, named for his father. Two things struck me, and they were difficult to reconcile. First, everyone looked as though they were having a good time. In each shot we all looked pretty and happy. I bought pretty— I didn't buy happy. And second, did I ever really inhabit that skinny little stick-figure body? I leaned forward and looked closely. There I was, all pinafores and braids. Oddly, there was something about me that didn't look quite American. I looked rather like the small girls I saw playing in a park a few years ago in St. Petersburg, Russia—I looked like an Eastern European child. Maybe it was those ribbon bows. It seemed as if, in those early years, my mother's Hungarian blood insinuated itself into the way in which I was dressed.

Were there any clues? Was there anything that indicated that that little girl could be me? But then, is there ever any indication? I've often stared hard at photographs of little children, trying to glimpse their later lives. That little girl in Denmark who became Isak Dinesen—is there anything about that Edwardian child in her prim dark dress that tells us she will journey to the Ngong Hills in Kenya and write of Africa as no one else ever has? Is it possible to see anything in the two-year-old Oscar Wilde, sitting on his mother's lap, that tells us of the dark road ahead leading him to Reading Gaol? And what of Sidonie-Gabrielle Colette? How can you possibly look at photographs of that thirteen-year-old girl in her sailor dress, braids to below her knees, and find the famous and infamous Colette—see that starting from there she would get to where she got?

I stared at the young girl on the screen. Somehow, because it was me I was looking at, I thought I should be able to see it, some hint of what lay ahead. I thought there should be at least one brief moment where something flickered across the screen, where I thought, *Ah, yes, there it is . . .* But I didn't—I glimpsed nothing. The little girl on the screen was a complete stranger to me.

CHAPTER 3

In the late eighties there was a woman named Ganga Stone who heard about one particular young man whose AIDS had weakened him to the point where he was more or less a prisoner starving in his own apartment. Ganga figured, quite rightly, that he probably was one of many who did not have the strength to feed themselves, and so she got on her bicycle, went around to local restaurants, and asked them to donate food, which she then delivered. Out of that experience she founded an organization called God's Love We Deliver, which has fed thousands of people with AIDS in all five New York boroughs. A great good was done as a result of her hearing about one particular man in one particular Upper West Side apartment.

Ganga and I used to compare notes. She told me that she could not live with the idea that someone was ill and hungry and not try to do something about it. I used to tell her that I could not live with the idea that someone was ill, frightened, alone, and not try to do something about it.

Here they were. All those young men, so very, very sick with a strange new most-likely-fatal illness that had no cure, that appeared to be sexually transmitted and had hit the gay community hard. It brought with it all the judgments and homophobia one might expect—in many cases there was little or no support from families and friends back home, and often, every friend they'd made in New York was just as sick as they were.

In New York City the artistic community was very hard hit—the world that was so important to me, the world in which we had so many friends. Then, too, my own relationship to death at that time was so fear filled I could not imagine anything more terrifying than to be a young gay man with the AIDS virus. This disaster had hit my world and my friends.

Then, as in Ganga's case, there was one young man who was the lightning rod—his name was Archie Harrison. Whatever may have prepared me over the years, and now I can look back and see that indeed many things had prepared me, it was Archie who opened my eyes, who showed me something I'd not known was possible—who changed my life.

The very first time I heard AIDS mentioned, it didn't yet have a name. I got a phone call from our friend "Bean." He told me that he'd not been feeling at all well and that his doctor was running a series of tests—there was some strange new illness in the land that seemed to be affecting only gay men, and the medical world was completely baffled. At that moment I was concerned for my friend but certainly not at all alarmed. I did not yet hear the distant beating of the drums.

In a very short time this new virus did have a name—Acquired Immune Deficiency Syndrome—AIDS. It was labeled an epidemic. New names of those who were infected were added to the list on a weekly basis. First you'd hear that someone had a bad cold that just wouldn't go away, then it was pneumonia, then it was PCP (*pneumocystis carinii* pneumonia), which meant it was AIDS. The reports, the predictions as to where this epidemic was headed, became darker and darker with each passing week. The media, with its fondness for the negative, scared everyone to death. There was real panic in those places that are more liberal and therefore have large gay communities—the big cities—primarily San Francisco and New York.

This crisis truly had my attention, and that's when I began hearing about a woman named Louise Hay who ran a support group in Los Angeles called the Hay Ride for people who were HIV positive. They met one evening each week, and word had it that the groups were encouraging and helpful and that there were tools to be gotten that were useful in helping people deal with the discovery that they were now living with a life-threatening virus for which there was no cure.

Ms. Hay had a very popular self-help book on the market which was all about how your thinking can heal your physical body. She was big on "affirmations"—standing in front of a mirror, looking yourself right in the eye, and telling yourself that you live in a strong healthy body free of disease. In 1987, I wasn't at all sure what I thought about her theories, but I knew that there were people with AIDS who were finding the work valuable and I was all for that, whatever it was. In the climate of dread created by the epidemic, if someone felt empowered by dancing in the moonlight with two chickens and a goat—I was for it. I was in 1987, and I am now.

That spring someone mentioned to me that Louise Hay would be coming to New York and doing a workshop in June. I'm not quite sure why when I heard the news I absolutely knew I had to sign up, but that was my reaction and that is what I did. Patrick, too, was a bit puzzled at that point as to what was going on with me. He was supportive but also curious, and I couldn't really explain it. Why was I spending my weekend in an AIDS-related workshop instead of hanging out with our boys, or going to the movies with him, or having people to dinner, or, or . . .

It was at that workshop that I first met Archie.

It was one of those workshops where we all sat on the carpeted floor of a hotel banquet room. It was not the first such floor I had sat on while attending a so-called self-help event designed to improve and enlighten. The carpets in such places are often covered with a variegated pattern designed to disguise spills and stains, which they do not do. That one consisted of geometric shapes in shades of brown and gray with a bit of deep wine red for color. I remember it perfectly—it was one of the uglier ones I'd ever seen. However, I did not go to the Days Inn Hotel on West Fifty-seventh Street at 9:00 on a Saturday morning in June to critique the decor. I was there because I wanted to be in a room with people who were living with such dire predictions about their mortality. I wanted to know how they were managing that. I wanted to hear what Louise Hay would say to them.

When I first arrived at the workshop there was a general restless-ness in the room. We had been instructed to bring a blanket and a pillow, and now people were shifting around, trying to get comfort-able, organizing their bit of turf. There were a few people already lying curled up on their blankets, clearly too weak to sit. There were many pairs of young men, often one taking care of the other. There were also other women in the room, most of whom appeared to be connected to one of the men—I was one of the few exceptions. Some people had brought backrests—I recall wishing I'd thought of that too.

The chatting in the room had been held to a soft whisper, then suddenly it stopped altogether as a woman of a certain age, followed by a small entourage of three or four very good-looking young men, came through the door and began threading her way among the people sitting on the floor as she headed for the low stage set up against the far wall. There was no question in anyone's mind: This was Louise Hay. She stepped up on the stage, turned toward her audience, and now everyone in the room was completely focused on her—this woman who was going to make things better. Ms. Hay was rail thin, had short-cropped bleached blond hair and artful makeup, and was wearing brilliant turquoise silk trousers and shirt—the sort of outfit one might wear to entertain on the patio. When she began to speak it was immediately apparent that she was a very com-manding presence. She began by outlining her theories on the ability of the mind to heal the body.

Oh, please, Louise Hay, save us! was palpable in the room.

When we came back from our lunch break I returned to my place, and now there was a young man lying next to my blanket whom I'd not seen before. He was beautiful—very thin and very pale, though because he had red hair his skin probably didn't have all that much color to begin with. His AIDS status was obvious. He was soundly and peacefully asleep. I was fascinated by him—couldn't take my eyes off him. After a few minutes I became aware that he was sleeping on the hard floor with no cushion. In a rush of pure instinct, I put my arm under his shoulders and lifted his head onto my lap. He opened his eyes, looked at me, grinned, and said, "Hi, I'm Archie," and then went back to sleep.

Late in the afternoon on the second day of the Louise Hay workshop, Archie was way across the room from me when he raised his hand and told everyone that for him the very hardest part about having AIDS was the fear that if he didn't make it, that if he died, he would be disappointing all those friends who were so vigorously cheering him on. All his friends were telling him he could do it—no matter what the dire predictions around this virus were, he could do it—he could be the miracle . . . and he didn't know if he could be a miracle. It just might be that he was going to die, and he worried terribly about letting his friends down.

At the next break, again on pure instinct, I went up to him and told him that I would dearly love to be his friend. I told him that it would be okay with me, that if he died he would not be letting me down, and that I would treasure whatever time we had together. Archie put his arms around me, buried his face in my shoulder, and wept.

At the close of the workshop Louise introduced two men, Robert Levithan and Samuel Kirschner, who'd told us about a support group for people who were infected themselves and also for the people who love them. This group, the Healing Circle, met every week in a music studio on West Fourteenth Street. Archie whispered to me that he would like to go.

At the very next Healing Circle there we were, Archie sitting in the middle with me on one side and his lover, Drew, on the other. Drew appeared to be healthy and strong, but I just assumed he was also infected. Turns out that's what he'd assumed too, but I found out later that at that point he had not actually been tested. He was already on overload with Archie's health and felt that was all he could handle right then, so he just kept putting it off. Also, he looked and felt perfectly fine and, as he told me later, there was probably the youthful invincibility factor in play as well. Drew did turn out to be positive, and he is now in a category called "elite non-progressor," which means that while he would still be classified as HIV positive, the virus is so weak at this point as to be almost meaningless. A perfect illustration of how very differently the virus behaves in different bodies.

This Healing Circle had a sort of anthem, a song they sang repeatedly, a song that had one particular phrase repeated over and over, "Spirit am I . . ." To look around that circle at all those young faces and listen to them sing about believing that their bodies were not who they were—spirit was who they truly were—these men whose physical bodies were failing them—both broke my heart and inspired. I remember that Archie sang with an amazing amount of gusto given his fragility.

That August, Patrick rented a boat for the month. He loved being on a boat—I like being on a boat when I know that it won't be too long before I can get off the boat. A thing we both loved was cruising around the island of Manhattan at the close of day, which is what we did one Friday evening with our two young sons, a group of friends including Archie and Drew, and several other members of

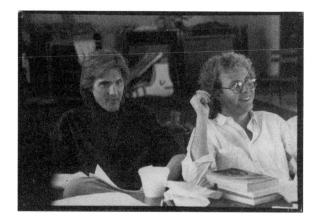

the Healing Circle. Out in the middle of the Hudson River, we were led in prayer by John Fletcher Harris, a Brit with a voice like Alan Rickman's. John blessed the river, the city, the sky, all of us, the entire planet and every creature on it. We sang "Spirit Am I" more than once. Then, as we were all hanging over the railing watching the city slowly light up—that most thrilling of sights—I looked at Archie's finely etched profile against the low setting sun. He appeared to be made of some thin translucent fabric, a fabric so thin it was as if the sunlight were shining right through him, and I knew in my gut that he was leaving soon, that he wouldn't be with us much longer. I didn't see how he could be—he was so frail, there was so little substance. I stood there on the deck, looking at him, asking myself, *Am I strong enough? Do I have what this takes? What the hell am I doing?*

A few days later Drew called me early in the morning—Archie had PCP pneumonia and was in Saint Clare's Hospital on intravenous antibiotics. I threw on some clothes and flew out the door.

Lord knows, visiting hospitals was a recent thing for me, and I'd definitely never been in one like Saint Clare's. At that time the neighborhood it was in, West Fifty-first Street and Ninth Avenue, was a pretty poor one—it hadn't been fancied up yet—and Saint Clare's was decidedly grim. I couldn't tell if it was really dirty or just so desperately in need of some fresh paint that it looked dirty. As I walked down the halls and glanced into the rooms on either side of me, I was very struck by what I saw: one bed after another in which a young man was lying—some asleep, some just staring into space. It's an old hospital, and the rooms are quite generous in size with unusually high ceilings, which made the single bed, the small nightstand next to it, and the one straight-backed wooden chair look even sadder and more forlorn than they might in a smaller room. That morning I did not see a single visitor in any of the rooms. What I was seeing was the visual manifestation of a reality—the reality that New York City was filled with young men with AIDS who had very little, if any, support around them. Focused as I was on Archie that day, I'm not sure how much it registered at the time. As the weeks went by I thought about them a lot, those visitorless rooms.

I got to Archie's room, and there was my darling friend in this depressing place, propped up on pillows, lines running into the veins of his right arm, smiling and happy to see me. Drew jumped up and gave me the one chair. With his very white skin and bright red hair, Archie looked like a small brilliant flame in all that sad grayness.

After Archie got out of the hospital and regained some strength, he once again threw himself into investigating every friend-recommended, alternative-healing modality in New York City. Just in the time I'd known him, besides the Healing Circle, he had meditated, prayed, had various forms of Eastern bodywork, bought healing oils, candles, shamanic artifacts, beads, crystals, feathers, and fetishes— he collected them all. He also put himself in the room with every spiritual teacher he heard about, and often I went with him. It was an education, much of it fascinating to me because most of the rooms were filled with people dealing with AIDS. The stakes were high. The issues and questions that came up were life-and-death ones—there weren't a lot of people wondering whether or not they should go with their boyfriend to Paris for the weekend. Some of the practices we heard about in those rooms were pretty extreme (drinking your own urine in order to save your life comes to mind), but if it doesn't look like you're going to be saved by medicine and science, you look for help elsewhere. I never for a moment sensed that Archie had any real fear of death, but he did love life and I did know he wanted to feel reasonably well and stay here as long as he possibly could. And oh, that was certainly what I wanted, too.

The extreme cold of that winter kept Archie mostly indoors. Given the fact that his lungs were obviously not very strong and he'd had pneumonia three times, he didn't want to risk any kind of chill or cold. He also worried about what other people might bring to him.

He questioned everyone about the state of their health before they visited. One day he snapped at Drew and me because we weren't washing our hands enough—we could be bringing in all sorts of dangerous germs! I couldn't help but wonder how much difference washing our hands could possibly make to the heartbreaking thing that was happening there in that room.

During that period at the end of the year, I saw Archie a bit less frequently; there was the cold, there were the holidays with my family, and there was a bad bout of bronchitis I'd had and didn't want to take to Archie. When I did go, he mostly wanted me to read to him. One day he handed me Christina Stead's *The Man Who Loved Children*, and that's what we began reading, one chapter per visit. It's a very long book, and with how frail he seemed, it was impossible not to wonder if we would finish it—a thought I constantly pushed aside.

As I was leaving one evening there was, as always, much hugging and kissing followed by a moment I will never forget. Archie looked into my eyes—straight into my eyes. Everything stopped. There was no time, no sound, no breath. In those long seconds we were absolutely connected—soul to soul. I felt as though this was Archie's real goodbye to me, as if with that intense look he was imprinting me so that I would never forget him—etching himself on the template of my memory.

When I met Archie in that first workshop, I thought he looked very fragile—which, of course, was nothing compared to the pale elegant ghost he became. It was as though he was slowly melting before my eyes—a front-yard snowman, diminished each time I looked out the window.

By the following spring Archie's physical problems became focused mainly in the gut; he simply wasn't able to keep down enough food to survive. Finally, after he struggled for many weeks, a decision was made to put a tube directly into his stomach. The first time I saw him after that was done, I was very unsettled by what I saw. Archie was lying on the bed, hooked up to shiny chrome machinery and plastic tubing, through which a thick off-white liquid dripped into his thin white body. He seemed so small on the bed—the machinery taking up far more space than he was—I couldn't quite find my friend.

The apartment that Archie and Drew lived in was a one-room West Fifties walk-up. There was a small bathroom and a tiny kitchen tucked into one corner. The whole thing was about as big as one of our two sons' bedrooms. Every time I went there I wondered how the hell they did it, these two tall men with their long arms and legs. I suspected that if Patrick and I had to live in such quarters, one of us would have murdered the other long ago. Now this little room was filled with all the necessary hardware and carton stacked upon carton of IV nutrients—claustrophobic and pretty damn depressing, but, as always, Archie seemed cheerful, optimistic, and very glad to see me. I'd say, "Hello, Mr. Harrison!" and he'd say, "Hello, Mrs. O'Neal!" Then we'd hug each other like mad. It occurred to me that I'd better find a way to be comfortable with that cramped little space—I'd probably be spending a lot of time there, as I didn't see how Archie was going to be getting around very much. It's not as though it was all bad—it wasn't. Being included in the lives of these two wonderful men who so obviously loved and respected each other—being trusted by them at such a profound time in their lives—watching Archie face the fading away of his life with such courage and grace: These were very great things. So I'd tell myself to pull up my socks and stop focusing on how small the room was.

One morning near the end of that July, Drew called and asked if I could stay with Archie for a couple of hours that afternoon while he went to work. I could. When I arrived around three, I was immediately struck by the fact that Archie looked sicker, even thinner and more ashen than the day before. When Drew left I climbed onto the bed and sat as close as I could get. We sat in silence for a few minutes, then Archie began talking. He told me that he'd been doing a lot of thinking and he needed my help. He wanted to stop the feedings and all his medications, except whatever he would need for pain. It had become clear to him that they were not working—he couldn't get enough nourishment to do more than just stay alive at the most minimal level of survival. Being hooked up to that machine all day was not a real life, and now he felt that it was time to let go. He told me that his spirit was strong but that his body was just too tired, too damaged, to go on. He also felt that if he unhooked everything and stopped all the meds, he could have some last days of real life—he could go to a museum for a final visit with his favorite paintings, he could go to a restaurant, a movie—in short, he could do the things he loved, one more time. He could also say good-bye to the people he loved. Then he'd leave us—his spirit would just fly off.

Next he asked if I would please stay with him while he told Drew. I said that of course I would.

Drew was magnificent—I don't know another word for it. He said that he would be all right, that he felt strong, and that Archie must do whatever he needed to do. He said this with eyes that were brimming with tears. I'd never been with someone who was urging the person they loved most in the word to leave them, if that's what was right for them. I'd also certainly never been with someone who was choosing death rather than wait for the moment when death could not be turned away.

At one point, when Drew was in the bathroom for a few minutes, Archie turned to me and said he knew that it was selfish but the truth was he wished that Drew and I could be with him every minute till the end—he knew that because I had a husband and young sons I wouldn't really be able to do that. I told him that I would be with him every moment that I possibly could—wondering as I said it how Patrick would feel about all of it. A little more talking and hugging, then it was time for me to leave the two of them alone.

A few minutes later, sitting on the steps of their building, I tried to gather myself for the walk to the nearest subway station and the ride home. As I sat there melting in the sweltering heat of that July evening, I thought about the fact that when I was in my teens, my passionate novel reading often included stories set in England against a background of the First World War. When I fantasized about myself as the heroine of these stories, it was not as the sock knitter, the bandage roller, it was as the young nurse in the ambulance driving furiously along the rutted French roads to get to the wounded young men in the trenches. In a very real way my fantasy seemed to be coming true, the AIDS epidemic had much the quality of a war—so many wonderful young men were dying, so many families were being called with the crushing news that their son was gone.

What had I done? I wasn't even sitting next to Archie when he told everyone in that workshop that he didn't know if he could survive this disease. When he said that and I got up and headed toward him, that's the stop-frame in the film, that's the moment I chose to change my life as I'd been living it up till then. Or anyway, that's how it seemed to me as I sat there, wondering if I could just pull myself together enough to get home and do the necessary shifting of gears required to be with my kids, greet my husband, and feed my family.

The next morning we were in the American Wing of the Metropolitan Museum, and Drew was pushing Archie's wheelchair from Sargent to Whistler to Sargent. I couldn't take my eyes off Archie's face. He was lit up with excitement and joy—looking up at the paintings, he was an excited kid, all fresh and scrubbed and happy. He'd completely transformed. Hooked up to that feeding tube and taking all those medications, he was sometimes disgruntled, and I even saw a whisper of self-pity from time to time. Now he was the open, full-of-life Archie I'd first met and fallen in love with. He kept saying, over and over, "This is such a wonderful day . . . a wonderful day!"

Archie was dressed in a lot of loose jersey—all his stick-figure body could bear. He was wearing a tomato red shirt, some turquoise jewelry, the bright green Indian corn necklace I'd brought him from New Mexico. With his red, red hair, he was a sight to behold—a bird of brilliant plumage. Many of our fellow museumgoers stared at him as we traveled from room to room, and I was sure it was not just because of how he was dressed. I kept wanting to say to people, *Yes, you're right—this is AIDS—this is what it looks like!*

That whole week was amazing. He went out a few other times, but for the most part Archie spent his time calling the people he loved and asking them to come over so he could say good-bye. His manner was exactly that of someone who was going off to live on the Amalfi Coast for a couple of years and simply wanted to spend a little time with the people he most cared about before he left. I watched people make their way out the door with tears in their eyes while Archie waved them off with smiles and gratitude for the part they had played in his life. I didn't understand how long it could possibly go on, even though almost nothing seemed to change. Since there was no flesh on him to begin with, I didn't really see any weight loss. He did seem to be developing a slight tremor, but that was the only sign of deterioration. He'd had nothing but a few sips of water that whole week. He appeared to be existing on pure spirit.

Then one day something very strange happened. I phoned him to solidify our plans for the next day—I was planning to go up in the afternoon to be with him while Drew did a few things in the outside world—but Archie said to me that it really wasn't necessary, he'd been wanting to do a little reading all by himself, he'd talk to me later. It wasn't so much the words—it was the coolness in his voice. I felt sick. Had I done something? What could it be? The one thought I had was that Archie might be getting to a place I'd seen in other young men shortly before their deaths—particularly the ones who had a strong spiritual practice. It was as though they'd begun to be far more interested in where they were going than in where they were. Perhaps

Archie's air of detachment was simply that, but still, I needed to know what Drew's take would be on why Archie would put off seeing me for the first time ever, what he thought was going on. But before I had a chance to do that, Drew called the next morning and said he thought Archie was dying and could I please come as quickly as possible. Within minutes I was pacing up and down the City Hall subway platform praying for the damn train to come and also praying that it never would. I was so frightened of what was happening, undone by the thought of losing Archie but also very fearful that I wouldn't be able to do whatever was needed. I was afraid that somehow, after all we'd been through together, I would fail my friends at this critical hour.

When I arrived Archie was lying on the bed surrounded by Drew and two other friends. He was in a very, very deep sleep—or was it a coma? I could see why Drew thought he was dying—that's what I thought too. At that time I knew next to nothing about the business of dying, but it was clear to me that some great shift had taken place.

A couple of hours later, as we stood around him, each with a hand on his cool white body, Archie suddenly opened his eyes, lifted his head from the pillow, and said, "I want some iced coffee, a Three Musketeers bar, and champagne!"

We ran to the deli next door and the liquor store down the street, then we were all back on the bed with champagne-filled glasses. Archie raised his glass and made a toast: "To my life!"

He drank most of the coffee, ate the candy in huge grinning bites, and drank all the champagne. Then, for the next hours, he drifted in and out of that bottomless deep sleep. His pulse was very slow, he felt cool to the touch. Now and again we spoke to him, reassured him that he was doing fine, that we loved him, that we were all right there with him. We told him to fly off whenever he was ready.

At one point he awoke for a few minutes, I asked him where he'd been, and he said he felt he had gone very, very far away. We joked that he was probably reserving a good room, getting things set up for his arrival with a tape player and armloads of peonies . . . As we'd been doing throughout, we massaged him with his favorite patchouli oil, candles were burning all around the room, and chamber music was playing. Everything was hushed—the room had become a sacred place.

As it neared midnight I could barely keep my own eyes open. I had to go home, kiss my sons and my husband, and get some sleep.

The next day was much the same—mostly Archie was in that deep comalike sleep. A few times he opened his eyes just long enough to smile at Drew and whisper a few words. Somehow, I'm not sure why, I just felt that things would stay as they were for many more hours—I was very tired and went home early.

August 8, 1988. I was on the subway platform again, waiting for the uptown train. I didn't know what I would find when I got there. I'd not talked to Drew since I'd left late afternoon the day before.

When I knocked on the door Drew opened it, looked at me with his sweet sorrowful face and said, "Well, he's gone—just a minute ago."

There was Archie, but not Archie, lying on the bed. As I looked at him I knew that in equal measure I'd known this moment was coming, and I'd also thought that he could never possibly die—not Archie.

We sat around his bed. I don't really know how much time passed. I was holding Archie's hand, which was becoming colder and colder each minute, more a piece of sculpture, less a human hand. We talked softly to each other and to him. The feeling in the room was gentle and matter-of-fact. There was no weeping or great emotion. We were all exhausted and numb.

I left before they came to take his body away—I couldn't be there for that.

A couple of days later Drew and I were careening down scorched, crowded August streets, screaming with laughter as we carried Archie's remains from the funeral parlor back to their apartment. We were laughing so hard we couldn't walk straight. They had put

Archie's ashes in a label-less shiny silver paint can! How could it be that our beloved Archie had ended up in a paint can? Oh my god!

Two of Archie's best friends, Lisa and Josh, hosted a lovely memorial service in their apartment. I was there but not really there, as I'd been all week since Archie died. My days had been hazy, unclear, and August hot.

Lisa and Josh's apartment was on the Lower East Side—it was charming, a bit funky, people filled, and un-air-conditioned. Drew spoke very beautifully and read from Archie's diary. I read the letter Archie's mother wrote to him after she got the news that he had contracted the virus, that he was HIV positive. It was difficult to read that letter around the great knot of tears in my throat. There were other words spoken, people talked with love and humor about that dear sweet red-haired man. There was laughter from time to time over wonderful goofy things that Archie had said or done.

Wine was poured, and we toasted him.

I drifted out.

I walked slowly across the city thinking about the fact that Archie had changed my life forever: that I had always thought that death was terrifying. I had thought that death was to be avoided at all cost, pushed way back in the corner of the attic where I didn't have to hear or speak of it; I had thought that death was eerie and menacing and I would never have the courage to be in the room with it. By demonstration Archie changed all that—every bit of it. Archie was not afraid of death, and here I had been thinking you had to be.

CHAPTER 4

Within the HIV community there was a constant trading of information—a new treatment, another doctor, a book that must be read, a lecturer, a seminar—which, of course, is how I met Archie and Drew in the first place. Whenever trying something new they almost always invited me to go along, and I almost always said yes. I was attending the Healing Circle every week and getting to know more and more people infected with the virus. This sweeping epidemic had engaged me in a way that nothing else ever had. I wanted to be of some help if I could just figure out how to do that. I wanted to know what to say. I wanted to know how to be with someone who was only twenty-one years old who'd been told they had, at most, two years to live—which is what, with very few exceptions, the doctors were saying.

In the fall before he died, Archie, Drew, and I sat in a church one evening listening to a woman named Marianne Williamson who, like Louise Hay, was a spiritual teacher based in Los Angeles. She also worked with the AIDS community and had created a place called the Los Angeles Center for Living, where people dealing with the HIV virus could go for a variety of services and, most important, where it was possible to talk about illness and death as natural parts of life instead of as a terrible failure or punishment.

Ms. Williamson's work was, and as far as I know still is, based on something called *A Course in Miracles*—she began almost every sentence with "As it says in the Course . . ." Here's where I was not so sure. The "Course" turned out to be a very hefty book containing material purportedly "channeled" through a psychology professor at Columbia University. This professor claimed that the voice speaking to her, whose words she recorded at the insistence of a fellow professor, was that of Jesus Christ. So the words this woman heard in her head and then put down on paper came with high credentials.

When we got to the church where Marianne Williamson was speaking, it was clear that a great many people had heard of her. It was well known that she was working with people infected with the virus and, as with Louise Hay, there was a powerful hunger to hang onto something in this threatening time. The church was packed, and Archie, Drew, and I were pretty well sardined into our pew. There was great excitement and anticipation in the air before Marianne arrived, and then when she did, I nearly fell out of my seat. I'd been in the presence of many spiritual teachers in the last decade or so, and generally speaking they had presented themselves wearing subdued colors, sometimes robes, sometimes shaved heads, that sort of thing. Not so this time. Marianne Williamson is a very pretty small, slender brunette, and that night she was wearing a brilliant red gabardine suit with a long jacket, the shoulders of which could easily have accommodated Fran Tarkenton, shoulder pads and all. The skirt hit about four inches above the ankle and was scalloped all around, having been gathered up in the manner of a Roman shade. This was topped off, or rather bottomed off, with red high heels and sheer red nylons that made her legs look as if they'd been boiled.

Once I adjusted to the visuals, I could see that Marianne was an extremely charismatic speaker—smart, quick, and very much in command. What followed—"As it says in the Course"—were for the most part principles I'd heard many times from many disciplines, principles that can be summed up by what it says in the Talmud: "We don't see things as they are, we see them as *we* are." Once again I was hearing that life is all perception. There was also a lot about prayer and meditation and love. All of that was familiar turf. What wasn't so familiar was what Marianne and the "Course" seemed to be saying about how things are only real if they are of love and God—and anything not of love and God doesn't even exist.

Afterward, walking toward the subway on that beautiful autumn night, I wasn't sure what I thought. For one thing, all the different spiritual teachings I'd been exposed to seemed to indicate that God was in *everything*—so what exactly were the things that didn't really exist according to *A Course in Miracles?* Was AIDS on that list? But that was not all Marianne said that night, and it was clear that Archie and Drew were smitten and immediately said they wanted to be there whenever Ms. Williamson came to New York. I did not speak of my reservations—I wanted to be nothing but encouraging about anything that Archie found helpful. I would go with them again because, for reasons I didn't even quite understand, I felt it was necessary to be with Archie every step of the journey, and it also seemed of the greatest importance that I be in those rooms filled with people facing AIDS and with the people who loved them. The pull to be involved with the crisis in a significant way was beginning to have a serious impact on my life.

After that night I tried to read *A Course in Miracles,* and I simply couldn't do it. I found the style, the syntax, very dense and awkward—for me it was just impossible. I'd read a couple of pages and then I'd find myself picking up *Anna Karenina* once again. I did much better with Marianne interpreting for me. At her third lecture in the church Marianne was focused on the power of prayer. She seemed to be saying that God will give you what you want if you just pray hard enough, just as Louise Hay seemed to say that you can have what you want if you affirm hard enough.

I am skeptical of such simplicity—the idea that it's possible to control life through prayer or affirming or chanting or anything else. What if you do those things with all your heart and soul and you still don't get what you want? What do you tell yourself then? You're not doing it right? You're a bad person? You don't deserve it? You're a failure? All this trying to change and fix things seems to me to be missing the point. To me the only thing that makes sense is to pray that I be given whatever it is I need to deal with whatever it is that shows up in my life—with as much skill and grace as possible.

I would have loved it not to be true, but I honestly didn't think that all the praying, affirming, or chanting in the world was going to save Archie's life.

I had been introduced to Marianne along the way, and one night after her lecture she said she wanted to talk to me about something and asked for my phone number. I was curious to say the least. Why would Marianne want to talk to me? I found out the next day. It seemed that Marianne thought there should be a Center for Living in New York—that given our enormous, ever-rising AIDS population, it was desperately needed. I agreed. I thought it was a great idea. Would I help her create such a place? A resounding *yes*: This would mean having in my life a real context within which to work with the AIDS community—Marianne's lectures were packed with people who were HIV positive—and it would be a way to be even more connected and hands-on than I already was. Also, with new cases diagnosed every day, it seemed to me to be desperately needed. Still, as I was saying yes, there was a little worm of worry nibbling away at the back of my mind: Working with someone as powerhouse as Marianne didn't necessarily look like a walk in the park, and I was going to have to see how I could manage my reservations about *A Course in Miracles*. If I had had my choice I'd have preferred a place where the work was simply holding to basic spiritual principles without promoting any particular doctrine—in other words, a place like Friends In Deed. But my excitement at being included in something so important overrode any reservations I had.

Marianne had clearly done some research: She knew I was married to Patrick O'Neal, knew I was connected to the theater community, knew we owned The Ginger Man restaurant at Lincoln Center, knew I knew people who could be of great help with such a project. All of the above is, of course, why she wanted to talk to me.

Marianne said that the first thing to be done was to raise seed money so that we could begin to look for a space to house the center.

The best way to do that would be to have a dinner and invite people who could, if so inclined, write checks. I immediately volunteered The Ginger Man.

I couldn't wait to tell Patrick, and when I did he was all for it—he thought it was a wonderful idea. He'd been watching me with some puzzlement all those months—all the hours spent with Archie, running to hospitals, my commitment to something outside our personal lives—all of it something he'd not seen before. He knew me well; it was obvious how important it was to me. Also, he had his own strong feelings about what was happening—his own world was being hit hard by the epidemic—a wonderful young actor he'd recently directed in a television movie had just been diagnosed and was dangerously ill. He said he would talk to his brother about our giving a dinner at The Ginger Man.

The next person I wanted to talk to was our friend, the director Mike Nichols—I wanted to know what he thought of the whole project and whether or not he would be willing to support it—would he come to the dinner? When I thought of people we knew who would understand the need for such a center, who would get the urgency of it all, and who were in a position to be of enormous help—the first person I thought of was Mike.

❖ ❖ ❖

Memory: Not long after we'd moved into the apartment with the butter yellow drapes, I was sitting up in bed reading one evening when I heard Patrick come in the front door and I heard other men's voices along with his. I thought all Patrick was doing was walking the dog and buying cigarettes—he seemed to have picked up some friends along the way.

When the three of them walked into the bedroom, I was absolutely amazed. One of the men Patrick ran into on his walk was Walter Beakel, a longtime friend of his—nothing so amazing there—

but the other was someone Patrick and I had watched on television just a few nights before. Mike Nichols and his partner Elaine May had performed on the *Ed Sullivan Show*. Nichols and May were a comedy team, unlike anything we'd ever seen before in our lives— sophisticated, intellectual, brilliantly funny, and like thousands of others we were completely dazzled. Now he was sitting on the edge of my bed chatting away.

Thank god, while I usually wore nothing at all or maybe an old T-shirt to sleep in, that night I happened to be wearing a very pretty nightgown. I was hoping Mike Nichols would think that's how I always went to bed.

❖ ❖ ❖

At lunch, over perfect plates of pasta, I told Mike about the project. I told him what I'd seen: the AIDS wards with the visitorless rooms, all the very young men, alone and frightened, the men who are so sick but don't have any support around them because all their friends have already died. I told him there were courageous supportive families, but there were also families who couldn't bring themselves to come to New York to be with their kids—they got the phone call telling them their son was gay and that he had AIDS, both things they hadn't known—and they simply could not face what was happening, it all was so frightening and so outside their known world. I told him all about Archie and his magnificent courage, how he seemed to have a deeply spiritual set of beliefs that resulted in his walking toward his own death without fear. I told him about Marianne's creating the Los Angeles Center for Living, how well it was working there, and how exciting it was that now she wanted to create a similar facility in New York. I told him how important I thought it was that we have a place here where we could support all those hundreds of young people who had little or no other support, a place where we could help them get to the kind of acceptance and peace that Archie had, a place where we could talk about that taboo subject—death.

As I talked, I was aware that I was not telling Mike everything, and I didn't feel great about that fact. I knew that if I told him about my concerns regarding being able to work well with Marianne Williamson, and certainly if I told him about *A Course in Miracles* and how AIDS didn't even really exist—I could just imagine the look on his face—that might well be the end of it. Certainly, I think of Mike as being a deeply spiritual human being but he prefers his spirituality on the pragmatic side—when things get a bit too New Age and woo-woo, he gets very edgy. I told myself those were things I would be able to manage when the time came, and they wouldn't get in the way of the greater good the center would do.

Mike listened very quietly to all I had to say, which in my excitement and zeal I said a lot. Then he said, "I've been feeling I had to do something but I haven't quite known what to do. Now I know. Thank you."

The Ginger Man dinner was a great success. The room looked beautiful, the food was excellent, and there were round tables filled with the rich and famous. Louise Hay came, and both she and Marianne spoke most eloquently about the crisis and the need for such a center. By the end of the night we'd raised a lot of money—enough to go out and start looking for a space. Before the dinner Marianne and Louise called for a prayer/affirmation circle, in which I, of course, felt obliged to participate. I stood there, holding hands, feeling uncomfortable and slightly foolish—wishing I could just run and disappear. But, that aside, it was a triumphant evening.

We found a space on Broadway north of Houston in the area of New York known as NoHo. Some work had to be done before we could move in. While that was going on, Marianne had begun coming to New York more often to work on what would become the Manhattan Center for Living (MCFL) and also to lead HIV/AIDS support groups. Temporarily the groups were being held in her friend Bruce Bierman's apartment. At those groups she announced our plans for the center —those were the people who would be the basis of our clientele.

I was truly excited about the project, yet there were still those particular aspects I was struggling with. I remember a night when Marianne did not get to Bruce's apartment on time because her plane was late. The room was filled with people milling around, waiting. As the minutes went by it became uncomfortable, one could sense the impatience in the room, and finally someone said to me that they thought maybe I should at least start the opening prayer. My reaction was to say, "Let's wait a few more minutes," and then I went to the bathroom and stayed there. Hid out.

Though the suggestion that I lead a prayer for that big group of people terrified me—I didn't lead prayers, that wasn't something I knew how to do, and I was very ambivalent about that whole part of things—while in the bathroom I was most definitely praying that Marianne would walk in the door before anyone found me. She did—not one of my finer moments.

After the group I overheard Marianne talking to the parents of a young man I'd visited at Saint Vincent's that morning. His name was Kevin. He couldn't have weighed more than one hundred pounds, though I'm sure he was close to six feet tall, and his body and face were covered with dark Karposi's sarcoma lesions. He was so weak he could barely speak or lift his hand from the bed. That darling young man was most definitely leaving this world very soon. I heard Marianne telling his anguished parents the business about how the "Course" says that things not of love and God aren't even real and therefore since AIDS . . . The looks on the faces of those parents were quite something to see. In those instances I didn't understand what the hell Marianne was thinking, and I wondered how I was going to work with her over the long haul. Then I reminded myself that once we were settled in New York, she would only be coming to town once a month, that for those couple of days it could all be navigated, and the rest of us would not be telling people at the center that AIDS did not exist. Also, so much else that Marianne said was incredibly helpful and empowering for this frightened community. At that time I absolutely thought that the bottom line was that Marianne Williamson was doing an enormous amount of good—I'd just have to button up and manage the parts that made me so uncomfortable.

When I was a kid, I went to Saint Matthew's Episcopal Church in San Mateo because that's where all good children went. What I heard there obviously had no great resonance for me because the whole business of going to church did not stick. Then, many years later when following Patrick's lead, I started attending talks and workshops with various spiritual teachers. I began hearing the principles of various Eastern disciplines, which for me had great resonance. When I heard the Dalai Lama had been asked what his religion was and he replied, "Kindness," I thought, *Ah, yes, there it is. That's it.* Similarly, in a book about the Buddha, I read that when asked by his students what he was—was he a saint, a guru, a master, a teacher, what exactly was he?—Buddha replied, "I am awake." These ideas made sense to me. Hearing that we are something far greater than our physical bodies, that what we are is spirit and spirit cannot die, made complete sense to me. Here were principles I could work with. Concepts regarding "virgin births" and "sinners" made no sense to me, nor did the idea that AIDS did not exist because it was not of God.

I had never worked in an office in all my life and was sure I never would—now there I was at a desk in an office five days a week. Originally Marianne invited me to be on the board of the center and I accepted, but then as we proceeded, it became clearer and clearer to me that that wasn't enough. I wanted to be hands-on, I wanted to work with the clients every day, so I told her I thought I should be the program director and that in my travels I had met all sorts of practitioners of the healing arts—therapists and bodyworkers, nutritionists and meditation teachers, and so on. I was sure I could get wonderful people to volunteer their time, and I could put together a full week of different healing disciplines. Also, of course, I would be on the spot—ready to talk to whomever walked in the door, ready to run to a home or hospital when someone was in crisis. Marianne agreed to give me the job but, when I think back on that conversation, there was something about her response that was less than enthusiastic. I think she would have preferred that I just stay on the board. However, on my side, I was so eager to get to work that I ignored the moment of silence, the look that flashed across her face, and simply charged ahead.

We quickly saw that it was most definitely not enough to have only one big AIDS support group a month when Marianne was in town. Clearly there should be one every week. So, after a short time, it was decided that three of us, two of the counselors and I, would each do one a month.

The night I led my first group I was absolutely scared to death, and I certainly had no idea it would turn out to be the first of hundreds of such nights. By now I had watched Marianne lead many, many groups; I had watched the ease with which she could handle anything that came up—deal with any challenge. She had *A Course in Miracles* down cold, she could go right to the place in the text that addressed the question, whatever it was. I could not. However, while I didn't have the "Course" under my belt, I did have hundreds of Al-Anon meetings. I did have countless hours spent with great spiritual teachers, including Ram Dass, Stephen Levine, Werner Erhard, and Baba Muktananda, but still I was sick at the thought that someone would bring up something that would completely throw me and I would stand there, fumbling for a response, looking like an incompetent fool, being of no real help to anyone. These were, after all, people who were used to the polished, professional, smooth-as-glass Marianne Williamson.

Walking to the front of that oh-so-crowded room that night required as much courage as anything I'd ever done in my whole life, maybe more. There must have been a hundred faces all turned, looking at me. Now I was the person to whom they were silently saying, *Please help me!* Many were faces I knew, many I'd never seen before. Marianne always began with a guided meditation; I began with a silent meditation—it seemed safer—I was definitely going to have to work my way up to guided meditations and prayers.

After the group, people came up to me and talked as though everything were all right, asked a question they'd been shy about asking in front of the whole group, or thanked me for something I'd said that they found useful—so I guess I got away with it. Still, I did wonder what the hell I thought I was doing. My education for the role I had taken on was the epitome of on-the-job training. I can remember a million mistakes I made, and I'm sure there were a million more I don't remember or didn't even recognize at the time. Often a specific moment from those days will flash before my eyes that still makes me wince.

One of the clients at the center, from the very beginning, was a literature professor named George, whom we had watched get progressively weaker and more fragile each time we saw him. He was a lovely poetry-writing man; we had many long talks, and I felt we had become friends. He had a young partner, Jack, who called one day, very distraught, to say that George was terribly ill and could I come over.

While visiting ill clients, I had now been in a lot of New York apartments, the likes of which I had never seen before in all my New York years. George and Jack's apartment was one such place. First of all, it was tiny. As with Archie and Drew, it was hard to imagine how two grown men managed to live together in such a small space. But, besides that, it was the spirit-breaking dirt and mess: sink and counters piled high with dirty dishes, clothes and papers everywhere, and dear George passing his final hours on a bed with tangled sheets that looked as though they'd not been changed in a month. It was certainly not the first such place I'd seen, but it always shocked me. These men came into the center nicely dressed, looking quite pulled together, and then I would see their apartments, the way they lived. I had to work hard not to let them see the dismay I felt.

George must have been a client of God's Love We Deliver because when I arrived, Ganga Stone was already there. At that point she'd had more experience with all of it than I and certainly had far greater wisdom. George was unconscious, his body continually moving around on the bed, and the smell coming off that bed was not easy to be with. I joined her and Jack—each of us with our hands gently resting on a different part of George's body, assuring him that we were right there with him, encouraging him to leave when he was ready to go.

At one point, I turned to them and referred to George in the third person. Ganga immediately took me aside and very kindly told me I must not do that—she said, "George is still here and it's important that we treat him with the greatest respect—though he appears to be unconscious, he is still an aware human being, and we must treat him with honor and not talk about him as though he's not present."

I was mortified, I felt so stupid and clumsy. Of course, those are the kinds of errors I so did not want to make. This world I'd chosen to be a part of demanded that I be awake every single moment. I judged myself hard for that bit of unconsciousness.

When the center had been open for a year, I was feeling good about what we were accomplishing—we all were. New clients came through the doors every day. The support groups were powerful and well attended. We had attracted amazing volunteers who brought us their skills and their open hearts. We were definitely putting love, support, and compassion into the lives of a great many very ill people who often didn't seem to find it anywhere else. We held a lot of hands at a lot of bedsides. We attended a memorial service a week. The AIDS epidemic raged on.

After about a year and a half Marianne came to town for her monthly visit and told us that while the work of the center was going well, the money and business aspects were not—it was all pretty much of a mess—so she had decided that what the place needed was an executive director. The rest of us thought all we really needed was a crack bookkeeper, but Marianne had recently read a book about the proper setting up of nonprofit organizations that stated that an executive director was all important, so she was now full-throttle on finding such a person. She would put the word out and then interview candidates when she came to town the next month.

An executive director was hired, and I was immediately very skeptical. So was my closest fellow staff member, John Juska. The center, above all, needed to be a quiet, calm environment—this woman was wired and edgy. She talked too much.

Each day when I walked in, I dreaded it a little bit more than I had the day before. In a very short time our new executive director and I were crossing swords on an almost daily basis. She had ideas for all sorts of changes that really could destroy everything we'd established. For one, she wanted to begin charging for some of our services, which would immediately have meant that some people would no longer be able to come. We had to be available to help everyone—that was the whole point. The truth was she didn't get it—she just didn't understand the work or the spirit of the place. Soon I found myself going in to work a little earlier each day so that by the time she arrived around 11:30, I'd done most of my desk work and I could just leave to spend the afternoon visiting hospitals. There was a tension in the place that made it difficult for me to even think straight.

Finally the inevitable happened. It was a Wednesday, and our executive director was the quietest I'd ever seen her. She spent the entire day in her cubicle, on her computer. When I finished facilitating the group that night, I went back to my desk and found the letter she had been working on all day. The letter listed my many sins, put me on probation, and said that my performance would be monitored on a weekly basis.

I didn't think so.

It took me less than an hour to clear my desk of my personal belongings and write a letter of resignation to Marianne and the rest of the board. My letter was short and to the point—I simply said that most regrettably I could not work with the new order of things. I also made one request: I asked that because my connection to the clients was such a profound one, I be allowed to continue facilitating the Wednesday-night groups, which I would happily do as a volunteer.

When I woke the next morning, it was hard to believe I wouldn't be going to the center that day, hard to believe my life had changed so radically, so quickly. Not seeing the clients every day was certainly the most painful part but, while I felt terrible that the place I'd loved so much was all coming unraveled, I must admit there was also great relief. I'd certainly not been happy there for quite a while. My promise to myself was that I would never again put myself in a place where I dreaded going to work.

When I got home that night, Patrick was wonderful—he reminded me that my connection with the AIDS community was so strong that even if the form changed, the work that meant so much to me could continue. For example, it would not be hard to spend a whole day just in the AIDS unit at Saint Vincent's, and that was exactly how I spent my first out-of-work afternoon.

John Juska called the next morning. I told him that a mean-spirited part of me wished he would walk out too. He said that was absolutely his instinct, but he knew that if he did the clients wouldn't have anyone there for them who really understood the work and, as much as he would like to, he didn't see how he could leave. He was right.

One by one, most of the board members called to tell me they were going to resign as well—they didn't want to be involved if I wasn't there. Also, I heard that the clients were signing a petition to Marianne requesting that I be allowed to continue facilitating the Wednesday-night groups when she wasn't in town. All this was most appreciated, but it did not change what a very sad business it was.

With his fine sense of timing, Mike Nichols called that morning—just checking in, wanting to know how things were going.

"Funny you should ask. Let me tell you what just happened . . ."

"Well then, fuck it—we'll start another one!"

"Are you serious?"

"Sure. With what's going on, there can't be enough of such places in this city. It's not about competition, it's simply about adding more support."

"Well, that's a great suggestion, but I can't even think about it right now."

"You don't have to. Take your time."

Feeling displaced and disoriented, I decided that a short trip to New Mexico would be a good thing—the perfect place to regain my equilibrium—the perfect place to look at what had happened and see what I needed to see, learn what I needed to learn. In New York the phone was ringing all day with calls from people wanting to talk about it. Those calls pretty consistently made me right and other people wrong—not particularly healthy nor good for me. I needed to think quietly about what I could have done differently, and while I was already coming up with some answers to that question, I was also beginning to suspect that what I first thought of as a disaster might not be a bad thing—quite the contrary. I told myself that there was plenty of time to figure out the future after I got back to New York, that I could just put all of it out of my mind till I returned—but it was mighty difficult not to think about that call from Mike.

Those few days in New Mexico were medicinal. There is nothing I love more than just walking and looking at mountains in the far distance—for some reason mountains soothe my spirit like nothing else, as the sea did Patrick's. The taller, the more jaggedly fierce, the better.

❖ ❖ ❖

Memory: I'm lying on my stomach on the living room floor coloring in a coloring book and listening to *Jack Armstrong, the All-American Boy* on the radio. My mother's in the kitchen cooking and my brother Robby is there with her, doing something that's driving her crazy. I've already heard her say, "Robby, stop it!" about a hundred times.

I'm waiting for Pawnee to get home. I always go out to meet him when I hear his car in the driveway. After he hugs me and asks me how I am, we walk very slowly back to the house, and lots of times he stops in the middle of the lawn and just stands there with his hands in his pockets, looking across the valley to the San Gabriel Mountains. At dinnertime the mountains are mostly the color of the violet crayon in my Crayola box. I always stand right next to him. Sometimes he says, "Oh, how I love those mountains . . ." I love them, too.

✧ ✧ ✧

On a Tuesday night, six months after resigning from the MCFL, I facilitated our first Big Group at Friends In Deed.

The meeting was lit by votive candles because we were still in the middle of construction, there were piles of lumber and electrical cable everywhere, we probably inhaled more sawdust than was good for any of us, but everything about it felt right—it felt as thought we were home.

This whole project, enormous and financially risky as it was, had come together with amazing ease—the kind of ease that makes you feel you must be doing the right thing.

When I got back from Santa Fe and called Mike to see where he was now regarding the whole venture, he was exactly where he had been when I left town—absolutely committed and ready to go.

This time we didn't need to have a fund-raising dinner in order to raise the seed money—Mike simply picked up the phone and began calling good friends, and in a very short time we had the money to begin. I called my friend Susan Penzner, who is a first-rate downtown real estate broker, and she asked me to tell her exactly what the space needed to be. I told her, and she said, "I know where it is." Mike and I looked at it the next day, and she was exactly right. It was the ideal space. Again we were on Broadway but this time down below Houston in SoHo. We even had (and still have) the blessings of a landlord who is compassionate about the work we do and said he would be honored to have us in his building. (I remembered a building owner Marianne and I talked to who told us that the people in his building wouldn't want to be in the elevator with people who had AIDS!) A famous interior designer, Bob Patino, heard what we were doing and said that he felt a strong need to give back to his community and that he would like to design Friends as a gift. We assembled a wonderful board of directors, and at our first meeting, Mike thought of the name: "Friends In Deed." Perfect.

How different it was this time. Or maybe the real point is how different *I* was this time. When we began the MCFL, I was very excited but also uneasy about certain aspects of what was happening, and I was completely inexperienced—scrambling like mad to learn what I had to know in order to do what was required of me. Now I had more than two years of experience, two years of learning what to do and, equally important, what not to do. Marianne gave me that opportunity, for which I will always be enormously grateful.

When I knew for certain that we were going to create a new AIDS organization, I called John Juska and invited him to lunch with the goal of persuading him to join us. I really didn't see how to do it without John, we had worked so well together, we were so of a same mind about the work. I didn't need to do a lot of convincing. The minute we sat down, John told me he was leaving MCFL, it was all going so wrong, and he was simply too unhappy there. "Well," I said, "Guess what!"

We then had a long talk about what we saw that had worked and what we saw that hadn't worked: Friends In Deed was going to be built on what we knew did work. We knew that sometimes we would be wrong about that, mistakes would be made, but the complete alignment of everyone involved was a strong place to begin.

So on that Tuesday night in September of 1991, I facilitated our very first Big Group. Already many clients we knew from MCFL were there—we said over and over that this was not a competition, we were simply adding more support to the community—this HIV virus was so fierce that there needed to be all the help and support there could possibly be. MCFL was on Wednesday nights, FID on Tuesday nights.

It was an enormous undertaking in every regard and, of course, with this new venture there was one great difference: Now I was where the buck stopped. As the Stephen Sondheim song says—I was excited *and* scared.

It was the fall of 1991 and there I was—director of a nonprofit organization, president of a board of directors, and facilitator of support groups for people with a life-threatening illness. Never in a million years would I have dreamed of occupying even one of those three roles—they all seemed unimaginably far from any life I had ever conceived. But consciously unplanned-for and surprising as it all was, there had actually been a true foretelling, which I had dismissed at the time.

One weekend, Archie, Drew, and I had gone to a workshop at which the subject of one's life's work came up. The seminar leader had talked about how important it was that people get up in the morning and spend the day working at something that inspired them, brought them joy. It soon became clear that not only were a great many people not doing any such thing, they didn't even have any idea what that work would be—they didn't know what they wanted to do. So the leader led us through a visualization designed to help people find their passion, that thing that would propel them out of bed in the morning, eager for the day ahead. I was immediately sure that the process would lead me to finding myself in some sort of light-filled atelier, a design studio, a costume fitting room, something of that sort. We closed our eyes, were led through a brief centering meditation, and the exercise began.

The visualization started with our waking in the morning. We were simply to notice the room we were in, to look carefully at the details, to get out of bed, get dressed, pay attention to what clothing we were putting on, and so forth. Throughout we were reminded that this day was the most perfect day—a day of our true heart's desire.

When I, figuratively speaking, opened my eyes, I found myself in a room I had never seen before—at least not in this lifetime. It was a corner bedroom in what was clearly a very grand house. It was large, high-ceilinged, the predominant colors were white and the dark reddish brown of gleaming wood. The casement windows were partly open, the day was fine, and long soft transparent white curtains were blowing gently. I immediately knew that I was not in a city, that I was way out in the country with miles of open space all around me. As I lay looking around the room from my beautiful big lacy bed, I could feel great excitement and anticipation for the day ahead. I remember that I had a moment of thinking that this was a very odd start to a day that would surely be about design of one kind or another—and where was New York City?

In order to get dressed, I went to a large armoire and took out a beautiful simple linen shirt and a dark skirt, which I found to be floor length. Then I reached for and covered myself in a big flowered fringed shawl. At that moment I laughed. Of course! Since my early teens, I had been obsessed with the great Russian writers, so now there I was, in nineteenth-century Russia—not completely surprising.

When I left my bedroom I found myself in a large spacious hallway, which wrapped itself around an imposing staircase leading down to the entranceway. I had a sense of many rooms and that there were servants in the nether regions, but at that moment I was alone. I went down the front stairs, out the front door, crossed a deep porch, and down some steps to a waiting *troika*—a carriage with three horses and a driver. We headed for the city—St. Petersburg, I would think. We went through miles and miles of wheat fields where peasants were working, and the feeling was that both fields and "souls" had belonged to my family and now to me. Clearly I went right into the sensibility of the period.

The journey was long but the day was beautiful, and, too, I was sustained by my anticipation of what lay ahead—though at that point I had no idea what that was. I vividly remember that there was the moment when I could first see the onion domes of the city in the distance and the moment when the horse's hooves left the dirt road and struck the cobblestone streets.

We rode, taking many turns, into the heart of the city, and my excitement grew with each minute. Finally we drew up to a very imposing governmental-looking building. There were two or three men outside waiting for me. They helped me down from the carriage, and there followed much bowing and telling me how pleased they were that I was there. I assured them that I was the more pleased— though I still had no idea what I was so pleased about. Finally these gentlemen ushered me in through the impressive doorway and led me down long marble hallways, speaking to me as we went, softly and with great respect. At length we arrived at a pair of mahogany doors, which seemed magically to open inward, and I stepped into the room.

It was a large room with windows all along the far wall. Lovely gentle golden light poured in, illuminating a long rectangular table in the center. On all sides of the table sat men wearing rather formal suits, apparently gathered for some very serious business. They all rose as I entered, and I was ushered to the one empty chair. As I crossed the room, my heart began beating faster and faster, and I knew that I was finally going to realize something I had wanted for a long time. When I reached the table, I greeted all the men and then began to seat myself. At that instant I knew clearly and precisely why I was there.

There was a war—we were meeting to discuss and make plans for turning my estate into a field hospital for wounded Russian soldiers.

CHAPTER 5

I think that my mother's life was a great disappointment to her—it was not at all what she'd had in mind, and certainly not what she wanted for me. There's a line in Tennessee Williams's *The Glass Menagerie* about going to the movies instead of moving. I think that's how my mother used books. There was definitely a yearning for another life that I always sensed in her, and I think she used her novel reading to take her to the places she'd never been and to which she would probably never go.

We always lived in a suburb—first Toluca Lake in the San Fernando Valley and then San Mateo on the San Francisco Peninsula. Though for most of my life I've thought that I am nothing like my mother, except for our mutual passion for books, I now see that living in those houses—with their neat yards and their streets on which an hour could go by without the passing of a single car, those streets on which no human being ever walked because they had no need to go farther than the car in the garage—must have deadened her soul with their lack of energy and aliveness, and that in that regard I am exactly like her. I could live in a small dusty western town with only my truck, my animals, a feed store, and a saloon and make it work. I know I could. But if for some unimaginable reason I were forced to live in some nice suburb, I suspect it would be about thirty-six hours before I was in a warm bath with a packet of razor blades. How did she do it, my mother who ached for a juicy life? Not only did she not have such a life for herself, she died just before I began to have exactly the life of her dreams. I've often been sad about that—I know that the early years of my married life would have given her great secondhand joy.

After I left school it was clear that I was not going to be handed any money by my family—to hear them, there was none to hand—therefore I needed to begin earning some on my own. Having no particular direction, no passion other then sitting about reading all day and night, nothing I was trained for, no real thoughts of a career—marriage was the career all my peers seemed to be focused on—so it seemed to me that the only asset I might have was my looks and that the only two places where one's looks had any real earning power were modeling and acting.

Without too much difficulty I began to get modeling jobs in San Francisco, doing runway shows and newspaper ads for the various local department stores in town. After about a year of this I decided—with the full support of my mother—that the next logical step was Hollywood, television, and movies. Moving to Hollywood would be allowed because, having lived in Southern California for several years, there were family friends who could keep an eye on me, or so my parents told themselves.

The fact that I had no training, had never studied theater in any way, shape, or form (unless you count the dramatic performances I put on for my boyfriends), that I had never even been moved to join the drama class in high school—none of this seemed a problem. I just assumed that as I had talked the necessary people at Saks Fifth Avenue into putting me into a fashion show when I'd had absolutely no experience on a catwalk, so I could talk someone into giving me a part in a television show or movie without my having had any experience. In truth that is more or less what happened. I spun a fanciful tale of belonging to some acting group in San Francisco, which got me an agent, who then sent me out on auditions. It wasn't too long before I read for a big part in a live television drama, and amazingly I got the part. So there I was—one full hour of *live* television when I'd never been in front of a camera before in my life. One thing I will say for myself—I had moxie!

In those early days of television, there were many live dramatic shows. One was called *Matinee Theatre*, and it was an hour-long show on every day at noon, Monday through Friday. Five dramatic shows each week created an enormous demand for scripts, directors, and actors. Often actors were flown in from New York for an episode. We rehearsed at the NBC rehearsal studios at the corner of Hollywood and Vine. At any given moment there were five shows being worked on in different rooms, all of which opened onto wide hallways with water coolers and pay phones where we, the actors, would take breaks during the long all-day rehearsals.

It was in these hallways that I met my first honest-to-god New York actor. In those days every young Hollywood actor was in awe of the Actors Studio and method acting. We had watched Marlon Brando scream for "Stella!" and say, "My name is Zapata, E-mi-li-a-no Za-pa-ta." We had seen Montgomery Clift look John Wayne right in the eye, saying, "My name's Garth. Matthew Garth," and search every millimeter of Elizabeth Taylor's gorgeous face with slow, passionate eyes. Then of course there was James Dean. Like everyone else I was truly, madly, deeply in love with all three.

One afternoon while working on one of the *Matinee Theatre* episodes, I went out into the hall to make a phone call. There was a young blond man (who turned out to be Steve McQueen) slouched against the wall in a posture that said, louder than any words, "Method actor!" As we were all alone in the hall and were coworkers of a sort, it seemed odd not to say something, so I said, "Hi," and he said, "Hi." I then made my call. As I passed him on the return trip, I heard some softly spoken, slightly slurred words coming from his direction.

"Hey—you dig men?"

"Uhh . . . yeah . . . sure . . ."

"Well, that's good, 'cause you're a real handsome chick!"

Now, I had never been called a "handsome chick" before, and while I sensed that there was a world in which that was probably a fine thing to be, as we talked further, with each short sentence followed by a very long, very intense pause, I could feel the tide pulling me out to sea. Also, inherent in his question was the notion that it might be possible to dig something other than men, which was a little advanced for me at that time. He was very sexy, and he intrigued the hell out of me, but I felt awkward and square. I didn't know how to talk his talk, and I was getting more uncomfortable and embarrassed by the moment. I told him I had to get back to my rehearsal.

I did more than a dozen *Matinee Theatres*, and while we were discussing the particulars of my contract for one of them, my agent at the time, Bill Robinson, told me that he had a client, an actor named Patrick O'Neal, who was a member of the Actors Studio and who was out from New York to do an episode that would go on camera a couple of days before mine. He thought we should meet. This O'Neal was a terrific actor and a great guy, and, well . . . he just thought that we should meet.

Bill came to the studios at Hollywood and Vine one afternoon to check on his two clients, and that's when he introduced me to Patrick. I remember the moment: We shook hands, I looked into Patrick's face, and there was a momentary stop-time. It was one of those moments that are rather like those visual puzzles where there's a drawing of a forest and you're challenged to find the chipmunk. At first you can't see the chipmunk at all, and then when you do, the chipmunk is all you can see. The chipmunk stands out, and the forest falls away. In the eye of memory that's how I saw Patrick. Everything else fell away.

I met Patrick O'Neal in June 1956, and we were married in January 1957. For every possible reason, nothing would ever be the same again. In those days it was most definitely not the norm to live together before you were married—I'm sure there were people who did, but I didn't know any of them, and certainly "nice" girls did not live with men they were not married to. So everything about living with a man, other than a father or a brother, was a brand-new experience.

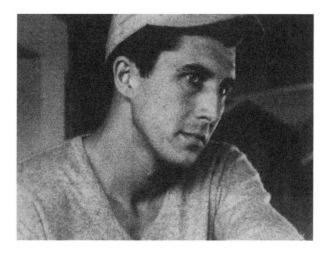

Then there was the matter of geography. I had always dreamed of going to New York City, and now Patrick and I were going to live in that glorious Oz-like city. I remember that friends in Hollywood could not believe I was leaving—here I was, a new young actor getting one good role after another—how could I walk away from that? Easy. Hell, the only reason I was in Hollywood doing television and having contract talks with studios was that I couldn't think of anything else to do. The money was good, there was glamour attached. I liked that, and my mother liked it more.

❖ ❖ ❖

Memory: There was only one telephone in our two-story San Mateo house. It sat on a table in the small central hall of the first floor. The voice of anyone talking on that phone floated right up the stairs, and all I had to do was step out of my bedroom to hear every word my

mother said. (On my calls I took the phone into the adjoining bathroom, snaked the wire under the door, sat on the floor, and
whispered.) Without her knowing it, I often listened to my mother
talking to her friends about me.

I heard, "She did a painting of flowers in art class, and it is so
beautiful! You know, Cynthia's just one of those people who excels at
everything she tries . . ."

I heard, "Well, of course she's the prettiest girl in her class, so naturally some of the other girls are envious . . ."

I heard, "This phone never stops ringing with boys from Stanford
wanting her to go out with them . . ."

Much of what I heard my mother say wasn't even true, but that
wasn't the worst of it. I had some tolerance for the notion that parents bragged about their kids. The worst of it was that there was no
pleasure for me in my mother's being proud of me. It never felt like
it had anything whatsoever to do with me—it was always all about
her.

❖   ❖   ❖

As it turned out, it would be more than a year before we actually lived
in New York City, before we moved into that beautiful West Village
parlor-floor apartment. Just as we began talking about getting married, Patrick was offered a television series that was to be filmed in
London, and so a beautiful little house just off Belgrave Square was
our first home together. If living in New York was exciting and exotic
to a California kid, living in London for a year was beyond anything
I could ever have imagined for myself.

Our pretty little house came with marble fireplaces, velvet sofas,
and a twice-a-week housekeeper named Mrs. Boor. The stairs
between the three floors were lined with emerald-green carpeting held
in place with a brass rod at the back of each stair. Once a week Mrs.
Boor would take each rod out of its bracket and polish it with brass

polish and a soft cloth till it gleamed. This was not a cleaning chore I had ever observed in Toluca Lake, San Mateo, or West Hollywood.

To fill my days while Patrick was at the studio, I went to the Cordon Bleu cooking school and signed up with a model agency, which resulted in my having photographs in London *Vogue* and *Harper's Bazaar* and all the other British fashion magazines. So, while I didn't know anyone in London, didn't really have any friends there, I did manage to stay busy until Patrick came home at the end of the day. I would cook some dish that I had just learned to make at the school, or we'd go out to a small local bistro and have a lovely dinner and a couple of glasses of wine.

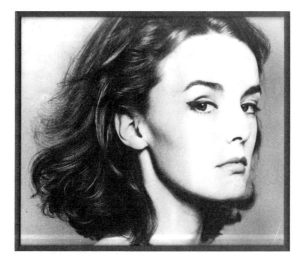

When the filming was over we stayed for another couple of months traveling around Europe. We wandered around great cities and beautiful small towns in France, Italy, and Spain. When I think about myself at that time I see that I was always working hard to appear sophisticated, as though a dinner at Maxim's were an everyday thing for me. For some reason I did not want Europeans to know I was really a girl from the Valley. Why that was so important to me I cannot say. Or maybe I can say. Perhaps it's something I learned at my mother's knee; I remember a conversation I once had with her half-sister, Betty, who told me that the problem with my mother was that she was always "putting on airs." It definitely wasn't something I learned from Pawnee. I once wrote him a letter about a wonderful elegant dinner we'd had in Seville, and he made fun of me with a report on a tuna sandwich he'd had in Redwood City.

✧   ✧   ✧

Memory: We arrived in London on January 18, 1957—just married and exhausted. At 7:00 the next morning, a car arrived to take Patrick to the studio where he would be doing his first day of work on the series *Dick and the Duchess*. He went off, and I was left alone in our hotel room at the Hyde Park Hotel. I had never been in a room like that before—never been in any room nearly so grand. The ceiling was way, way above me, encircled by miles of ornately carved moldings; the carpeting was thick and very beautiful; the pillows and bolsters and comforters on the bed must have used the feathers of ten thousand geese. In putting us there the producers of the TV series had certainly spared no expense. I recall wondering if it would have been any different if they hadn't known we had just gotten married.

I didn't tell Patrick that I was anxious about being left alone, but I was—very. The waiter who brought my breakfast was so superior to me in every regard he scared me to death. When I called room service to order breakfast, they asked me if I'd like a kipper. I said yes; I didn't know how to say no. I'd read about kippers in a hundred English novels, but when I tasted it I didn't see the charm of it and flushed most of it down the toilet. Then I guessed I should get dressed and get out of there because it seemed likely that another frightening person would come soon to make up the room.

I had no idea what to do or where to go.

❖ ❖ ❖

After more than a year of living in Europe, I arrived back in the United States with a few assets I'd not had when I left: I had a portfolio filled with photographs from various European fashion magazines, which got me working in New York City right away; I'd learned something about fine wine; I could make a very good *coquilles Saint-Jacques*; I could speak knowledgably about London theater; I could recommend marvelous little restaurants and shops in most of the major cities, ordering in French in French bistros and in Italian in Italian trattorias; I could sashay around the streets in high-heeled Chanel slingbacks, which hadn't quite arrived on our shores as yet, and a British racing green coat I'd bought in Paris that was so special people stopped me on the street, wanting to know where I'd gotten it.

CHAPTER 6

I grew up knowing about crisis. Crisis and I are old, old friends. Crisis has been hanging out with me ever since I can remember. I was only two years old when it first raised its terrifying ogre face. I don't think you're supposed to be able to remember something that happened at the age of two, but I most definitely remember this: I was in my high chair by the kitchen window and I began to cough and then choke. There was a strange sound coming out of me—I can hear it still. Now there is a gap in my memory but I clearly remember lying on a table with a blindingly bright light shining straight down on my face while some strange people with masks covering their noses and mouths put things down my throat. Even if I was far too young to understand exactly what was happening, I certainly sensed the fear that made my mother and father nearly crush me with their hugs in the hallway outside the operating room once it was over and I was out of danger. That experience made me understand in the deepest part of me that the world was not a safe place, terrible things can happen with no warning—my god, all I was doing was sitting in my high chair on a sunny California afternoon, having a little snack, and I was nearly lost.

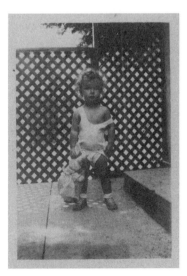

My parents had terrible fights:

Doors were slammed, dishes were broken, walls were punched. I now understand that my father was an alcoholic. Not that he drank all the time, but when he drank he completely transformed. My darling husband, who knew what he was talking about, used to say that *Dr. Jekyll and Mr. Hyde* was really the tale of an alcoholic, and that certainly described my father: Charming, funny, warm, affectionate, when sober Dr. Jekyll—one beer and Mr. Hyde emerged as an angry out-of-control nut case, so I was always afraid he would hurt my mother or my brother (he never actually did, and blessedly for me I was very rarely the object of his rage). I was also afraid that—and for me this was the most frightening part of all—he would go away and not come back. I adored my father.

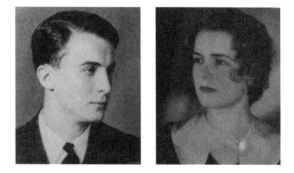

I adored him even though at times he scared me to death. The earliest Christmas season of which I have any memory contained two polar-opposite events. One evening my mother was standing in front of the bathroom mirror making up her beautiful face prior to going out—that most intriguing sight—and as I stood looking up, watching her, I began to recite "The Night Before Christmas." It had obviously been read to me a great many times because I was able to recite the entire thing, word for word, and I was only three years old. My parents went mad with delight. That was followed by another evening when my father and a friend of his sat around drinking, laughing, and shooting the ornaments off the Christmas tree. I have no idea what sort of weapon they used, but whatever it was it sent me to my room where I lay curled into a tight ball under the covers, listening to the popping sound of the glass ornaments shattering and the sound of my mother crying in her bedroom.

At those fear-filled, stomach-knotting times, my mother often sent me in to try to reason with my father. Once during a vacation (maybe the one when I was in that little rowboat showing off the tiny fish I'd caught), in the dark of night Pawnee was storming around the cabin, threatening to kill my brother if he didn't quiet down. My very little brother was having an asthma attack, and his crying and wheezing was keeping my father awake. My mother begged me to do something, to distract my father, make him laugh, use my adored-daughter charms on him—a heavy assignment for a seven-year-old.

Not every crisis was personal. December 7 fell on a weekend, and my father and I were in the backyard working in the garden when a friend of his, Gil Landau, came crashing out through the back door yelling, "The Japs have bombed Pearl Harbor!" (Yes, I know—but that *is* what he said—"The 'Japs' have bombed Pearl Harbor!") My father ran into the house, me right behind him, turned on the radio, and there it was. *War!*

Now crisis was in the air all around me, day and night. Japan was right across that ocean whose waves I often splashed about in on weekends. We were vulnerable. We were taught to get under our desks at school should the bombs start falling. We practiced blackouts—making sure that not a sliver of light could be seen between the curtains or drapes. Gas, meat, and butter were rationed—perhaps other things too that I don't remember. There were no nylon stockings—my mother put dark liquid makeup on her legs and then drew a line up the back with an eyebrow pencil to look like the seam that nylon stockings had in those days. It's what many women did during the war, and it fooled no one. The substitute for butter was a nasty white brick of some sort of lardlike substance that came with a pellet of yellow powder that had to be mashed into the white brick to make it look like butter. The mashing took a great deal of elbow grease, and the end result bore no relationship whatsoever to the real thing. We saved tinfoil from the linings of my parents' cigarette packages and rolled it into a shiny silver ball, which was then taken somewhere for something to do with the war effort. We had an enormous "victory garden" filled with every possible vegetable. My mother cut long strands of my then-blond hair and sent them off to be used for the "+" in bombsights—source of the expression "caught in the cross-hairs." (Years later I lay in bed one night horrified at that memory and thinking about the fact that targets may have been sighted with the help of my hair. and bombs dropped that killed people. It made me sick—I should have been asked if it was all right with me!) Soon flags appeared in the windows of the houses in our neighborhood. They were small white flags with red borders and stars in the middle—blue stars for the fathers and sons who were in the service—gold stars for those who had been killed.

Now we lived in a whole world of crisis. The war was all the adults talked about. They listened day and night to the news on the radio and had fierce arguments about what FDR and America should do. I think for me at that age it was somewhat frightening but also very exciting. I liked the heightened unusualness of everything, I liked the adrenaline, I liked the fact that almost nothing was the same. I also think it was probably some sort of relief to have a crisis that was outside my own home—that did not frighten me the way my father's rages and my parents' fights did. The war was a crisis that was in my life but at a comfortable remove. I had the talk and the drama but not actual war reality, until two things happened that did make that geographically distant war very real for a time.

The first, again, was on a weekend; my father was outside on a ladder cleaning leaves out of the rain gutters, my mother and I were in the kitchen doing the breakfast dishes. Suddenly there was a deafening crash that was so powerful that things flew off the counters and smashed on the floor, the dogs and cats skittered for cover, and Robby wailed from his playpen in the next room. In a few seconds my mother and I could see that we were still alive and all in one piece, but it seemed that the terrible impact of whatever it was had come right from where my father was. We tore out the front door and there he was lying unhurt in some bushes, having been knocked off the ladder, and there before our horrified eyes was a fighter plane buried to midwing in the roof of the house next door—just a small patch of grass, a flower bed, and a low picket fence away. The pilot was of course killed immediately, the plane and the house were in flames, there was the loud popping of bullets exploding in the intense heat, and fortunately the family that lived there was saved by the fact that they were out doing their weekend shopping. We later heard that the young pilot-in-training had been showing off fancy maneuvers to his girlfriend, who lived in the neighborhood. I remember my mother telling me that when you lived in a country where there was actually a war going on, such disasters could happen at any moment, day or night. That heartbreaking incident made the war very real for us.

My parents had a close friend, Mary Fowler, who joined the WACs (Women's Army Corps), attained an impressive rank, and was assigned to the nearby veterans' hospital. She invited us to come to the hospital for a tour of the facility, to see where she worked and what she did. My brother and I went with our mother, and we were barely inside the front door when I knew I was in terrible trouble. It took only a few seconds to see that there were soldiers everywhere—bandaged and broken; parts of them missing; some with scarred, burned, distorted flesh; some making their snail-paced way across the floor with canes and crutches. I can still see, as clear as day, the anguished face of one handsome young man with heavy bandages over both his eyes, feeling his way along the wall with both hands. I took the rest of the tour, holding tight to my mother's hand and staring straight down at my shiny black patent leather Mary Janes moving across the linoleum. Those images filled my head and my dreams for many, many months—I still recall them from time to time—and neither my brother nor I remember anyone ever talking to us about what we had seen. What on earth were the adults in my life thinking?

Following one horrific news report on the radio, I told my parents I knew that war was bad, that it was awful that so many people were dying, and that bombs and guns were terrible things, but I also thought it was kind of exciting. My parents didn't like that, and they told me that war was definitely not something to be "excited" by. I remember my father being particularly upset with me—the tense face of his anger was not often turned in my direction.

I think there was a way in which the war was helpful to me. It quieted some of my own anxiety. Given how long ago all this took place, it's difficult to remember the details, but I have a definite sense that the war drew my parents away from their personal conflicts; there was such intense focus on other parts of the world and on what decisions President Roosevelt was making that they seemed to have less energy for their own battles.

The death of a parent must be at the top of the list of all children's fears—the ultimate crisis. I assume this because, as a kid, the thing that frightened me more than anything else in the world was the thought that one of them would leave or that one of them would die.

❖   ❖   ❖

Memory: I was up in my second-floor bedroom in our house on Hurlingham Avenue in San Mateo, California. It was about ten o'clock at night, and I was sitting at my desk doing/not doing homework. I heard the phone ring, and I headed for the stairs. A call at that hour had to be a call for me.

I was halfway down the stairs when I heard my mother say hello.

A long silence. Then she said something so softly that I couldn't hear it. During the silence everything in the house shifted, held its breath, changed color. I froze midstairs.

Then I heard my mother hang up the phone.

"Ohhhh . . . My Bob . . ."

I ran to her and found her doubled over. She told me that my father had been in a head-on collision on El Camino Real as he was heading home from the city. She had to get to the hospital. She called our next-door neighbor, who said that he would drive her right away. I couldn't go with her. My brother was upstairs asleep. I had to stay there and wait for word of how bad it was. She'd call me as soon as she could. Waiting didn't seem possible.

Two unendurable hours later, the neighbor's son, my good friend Rae, called and told me that my father was in a coma but that he was going to live. When I answered the phone I was so demented with fear I didn't recognize Rae's voice, a voice I knew as well as anyone's in the world. My mother didn't come home until well after the sun was up.

During all the waiting hours, my head echoing, over and over, "Ohhh . . . My Bob . . ."

A tape on continuous play.

✧ ✧ ✧

It was many weeks before my father could go back to work, and his recovery at home was a turbulent, scary time. The injuries he sustained were all to his head, and they affected him in much the same way alcohol did. He was moody and full of anger and generally almost impossible to be around. It was especially hard on my mother, who was trying to take care of him. She told me that we had to understand that his accident was a terrible trauma, that he still loved us, and that he would be himself again one day soon. Of course "himself" included those dark humors anyway—just not all the time.

Then, not very long after my father was well enough to return to work, I was sitting in my sixth-grade classroom when the secretary to the school principal came in, went up to our teacher, whispered something to her, and then came over to me and told me that the principal wanted to see me in his office—already absolutely terrifying. What had I done? No one was called to the principal's office unless they were in serious trouble. As it turned out I wasn't in trouble, but my mother was.

I can still feel what it was like to be twelve years old, sitting in that office while the principal told me that I had to collect my younger brother and go right home—that my grandparents would be waiting—my mother was in the hospital. When Robby and I got home, I found out that my mother had had a stroke, that my father was with her at the hospital, and, again, I would be called when they knew how serious it was.

My grandparents were useless. My University of Breslau–educated, dueling-scarred grandfather sat in the chair he always sat in, imperiously drinking cups of tea that my grandmother made and served him when she wasn't running in circles and wringing her hands, saying, "Oh, my poor Bob! My poor Bob!" At one point I screamed at her, "What about my mother—*what about poor Helen?!*" My grandfather told me not to be rude.

My mother recovered from that stroke without any serious lasting damage of the kind that often accompanies strokes, but she was never completely herself again. She was always a bit "fragile" after that. In the next few years she had two more mild strokes—"mild," but enough to have me lying in my bed at night wondering if I was just a heartbeat away from being without my mother.

Ten years after the first stroke, in the early evening of April Fools' Day, she called me from her bedroom in a voice that was doing everything it could to stay calm—a voice that immediately told me something was dreadfully wrong. I raced into her room and found her lying on her bed holding her head. My father had just left to drive up to San Francisco. She said, "Your father was going to stop at Gil's on the way—call there and tell him to come home." I phoned the Landaus', where my father had just left. Then I called for an ambulance.

My brother and I were sitting side by side in the hospital waiting room when a doctor came out and told us that our mother was gone. He asked if we would like to see her. Neither of us had the courage for that.

Somewhere in my chaotic youth, I began to feel that trouble was my "lot." As I look over what I have just written about how my family seemed crazier and more disaster prone than any other family I knew, I realize that in truth there was something else that set my parents apart in my eyes. With all the negative things I saw about them, I also saw their passion. I saw a fight at night followed by my father bending my mother over the next morning's breakfast dishes in a long slow kiss. I didn't notice other parents doing things like that. I think I connected the dots and decided that good stuff comes with bad stuff—that you don't get one without the other. It seemed to me that drama and passion were probably in my genes and that I was not destined for a calm orderly life.

When I really look at it, I think crisis holds a real seduction for me, and certainly there is some magical thinking involved. I understand perfectly well that there is no deal-making with God, but that doesn't mean I don't still try. There's a primal place in me that thinks that if I do my very best to help other people in their crises, disaster will stay away from me and mine. No one needs to tell me that that's ridiculous. I know it is. But I think that, for so many reasons, the AIDS epidemic gave me something I'd been needing without even knowing it—it gave me a crisis with all the adrenaline-charge a crisis always has, it affected me personally because I had friends who were dying, yet my own immediate family would seem to be safe from it. In a terrible way it was perfect. There is a place in me that hopes that if there is the dark evil shape of crisis "out there," occupied elsewhere, there's a better chance that crisis will not trouble itself to come to my door.

CHAPTER 7

A mother, whose son had died the week before, came to the Big Group one night. Her son had been a client for several years; this was her first visit. She came with a goal, a very specific purpose. She wanted to persuade every young man in that room to tell their mothers the truth of their HIV status if they hadn't already done so. Her son had kept the fact that he had AIDS a secret until he was in the hospital, dying, and had no alternative but to tell his family. He hadn't told them because he didn't want to upset his mother. This mother was heartbreakingly eloquent about how painful that decision was for her. She felt excluded from her son's life—her son whom she loved more than anything in the world. She felt not trusted, and her son had deprived her of being able to do the very thing that mothers are born to do—take care of their children. Please, please, she said . . . tell your mothers, don't try to spare them—don't cut them out of your life.

I looked around the room as she spoke—all those mothers' sons—the deep listening on their faces.

The parents: At Friends In Deed we've heard about and seen every kind—from the most loving to those whose treatment of their child is, by any humane measure, downright cruel. We see parents who come running at the first hint of trouble; we've been told about those who, when they learned their child was gay, told them to get out of the house, they never wanted to see them again. I've been told more than once by sons and daughters who were nearing the end of their lives that it's better their parents aren't there—they don't really want them in the room. Imagine.

Thinking about it, I realize that we spend a good amount of Big Group time on the subject of parents. Our clients are in their twenties, thirties, forties, and above—and still they are fretting about what their mother said on the phone last night or some enraging thing their father did when they went home for Christmas. We see that while some have chosen not to see their parents or have any contact with them, it doesn't mean they don't think about them all the time.

There is a young man in the Big Group recently who spoke of his mother, who lives in the Midwest. She has been an alcoholic for almost all his life. She has been a very poor mother—really she has been almost no mother at all. Many times he has talked about having to cut off communication for a while because for him she's toxic—a conversation with his mother can wreck the next several days—yet he can't let go of her. He obsesses over every word she says, each shift in the tone of her voice. She drives him mad and always has. But as he spoke of the fact that his mother was now in the hospital, her health clearly deteriorating and broken as a result of her addictions, his eyes filled with tears, his voice trembled, and he had to fight hard for control. He so doesn't want this mother to leave him, even though she has rarely been able to demonstrate any real love for or nurturing of her son.

Many parents wish their child were different (which in many cases means they wish their child weren't gay)—they want a child who is not the child they have, and by the same token many clients want parents who are not the parents they have. They're doing exactly the same thing. When we point it out to them, that thought always seems to surprise.

After the impassioned mother made her case for telling mothers the truth, a client raised his hand and talked about his home life and the verbal and physical abuse he'd experienced from early childhood. He obviously wanted that good mother to hear that all parents are not like her—that there are families where you are constantly humiliated and where telling the truth would only buy more pain.

Walking home that night, I thought about my own sons. When they were little boys I assumed that when they were grown we would be connected and close, which thankfully we are, but it never occurred to me that I would still be so concerned about them that I would think about them a dozen times a day, yet that is exactly what I do. I think about them a dozen times a day. I am always quietly praying that they are safe. Perhaps, in my case, it's exacerbated by years of watching heartbreaking things happen to mothers' sons. Perhaps I live in a world where I am constantly reminded that children can die before their parents—that most unbearable of all thoughts. Not only is it possible, it happens all the time. Were I in some other life, some other work, I would do my best to avoid such thoughts. But here at Friends In Deed, the thought cannot be hidden away. It is always there, floating at the edge of my consciousness, even when it's not right before my eyes.

At our next staff meeting we talked about the broken-hearted mother who took the time to come to a place she'd never been before to plead her case on behalf of mothers. That led to a general discussion of families and how they treat their HIV-infected sons or daughters, and from that to talking about some generalities we've observed over the years: one being that we most often hear of unloving homophobic prejudice coming from families in small towns in the middle and the south of the country—certainly most strongly from religious-right families. Ignorance is rampant. Based on what we have heard from hundreds of young men and women, this country is populated by a great many people who still think that homosexuality is a "choice," despite all scientific evidence to the contrary. I once had a fine lovely young man tell me that he knew he was an "abomination." That's what his Christian religion had taught him. Somehow I don't think Jesus Christ would have endorsed that particular point of view, but that is what is being taught at many churches in the land, and we often have to deal with the fallout. It's very difficult to put together a rich valuable life if you see yourself as an "abomination"—"abominations" don't deserve happiness. That particular young man also told me that he knew full well that he was gay when he was five years old—clearly he got an early start on becoming a loathsome sinner. I have fantasies of tearing into those churches on a Sunday morning, racing up to the pulpit, and setting those closed-minded bigoted fools straight—knowing, of course, that the chances of my being able to accomplish any such thing are mighty slim. I said it was a fantasy.

Another generality, one that I hadn't really been aware of before the AIDS epidemic, is the particularly harsh intolerance of Latino fathers toward gay sons. Having a son who is a top-of-the-line macho guy seems to mean the world to most Latino fathers, and we have met many sons who sadly haven't spoken to their fathers in years. From the sampling we see at Friends In Deed, I would guess that New York City is filled with young Latino men who moved here in great part to hide their sexuality from their families in whatever Latino country they come from. We've heard many accounts of hurriedly hiding the HIV meds and stashing all the photographs of beautiful scantily clad young men under the mattress when the family was coming to visit.

One of the most disturbing portraits of a Latino father was painted by one of our South American clients. When he first arrived, he told us his name was João, but since most Americans don't pronounce it correctly, he said we could just call him John. We said that there are a lot of "Johns" around FID, so given his place of birth we'd call him "Brazilian John." That idea split his face into an enormous grin.

Brazilian John was small, dark, and somewhat fierce looking—the bandit Joaquin Murrieta without the black cape. He was very smart. His English was excellent, and he was fluent in three other languages as well. He said that he was always at the top of his class—he had to be, because if his marks weren't perfect he would be severely beaten by his father. Whenever he raised his hand in Group, which he almost always did, somewhere in what he had to say would be something about his family and how he never wanted to see them again; he wanted nothing to do with them but, once more, he couldn't stop talking about them. His description of his father and the beatings he received made Benito Mussolini look like a pussycat, and his anger toward his mother was almost as intense—she never did one single thing to protect him. He had cut them off completely. They were no longer his family—Friends In Deed was now his family.

His Brazilian family did not know he was gay. His Brazilian family did not know he had AIDS. One day he told me, in private, that if his father ever knew his son was gay, he would come to New York and kill him.

Brazilian John was as courageous as any client we've ever had. One night in the Big Group he told us that he'd been diagnosed with AIDS-related CMV retinitis (which can result in total blindness), but it wasn't really a problem because, loving animals as he did, he'd just get a seeing-eye dog and that would be wonderful—the most wonderful thing in the world!

He lived in New Jersey, came to Manhattan each day on the PATH train, and when he got off the train he'd put on his Rollerblades and go tearing along like the wind. His favorite garb, in anything but the most freezing weather, was a pair of very short shorts and an undershirt that exposed a good expanse of chest— including the part where his Hickman catheter was embedded. A Hickman is a thin flexible tube inserted into a vein or blood vessel near the heart, which has an opening or two through which blood samples can be taken or medications given—most people who have them are extremely sensitive about them. I know guys who spent a whole summer at the beach without ever taking off their shirts, so sensitive were they—a Hickman screams out that you have AIDS. None of this was a problem for Brazilian John—he displayed his Hickman like a Purple Heart—even a Medal of Honor. So flying along the streets he'd go, straight black hair flying, Hickman exposed, grinning like crazy! Sometimes he arrived with his pet ferret in his knapsack. When he opened the knapsack the ferret would jump out and run about, cowering in various corners. To me he never looked like a very happy little creature, but then I'm no expert on the moods of ferrets. He was just about as wonderfully eccentric as anyone we have ever had come through our door—Brazilian John, not the ferret.

After he'd been with us for several months, we began to worry about Brazilian John's medical support. He'd been saying that his New Jersey doctors were perfectly fine and that he was doing well, but that's not how it looked to us. His color wasn't normal, his physical energy was visibly down, and then one day he limped in admitting that he felt like hell and that his doctors didn't seem to know what to do anymore. I immediately went to the phone and called Dr. Paul Bellman, the AIDS specialist with whom Friends In Deed has the strongest connection. I told him about Brazilian John, and he knew right away exactly whom I was talking about. He'd seen him Rollerblading around the downtown streets, saw what a courageous survivor he was, and told us to send him right over. We all sighed with relief. We have watched Dr. Bellman pull people back from the edge of the cliff time and again. Please god, he could do it again this time.

Brazilian John improved markedly under Bellman's care. He began showing up every day looking like his old energetic self. Whenever he was at Friends, he insisted on cleaning everything in sight, so we decided to make it official and gave him the job of Friends In Deed's "housekeeper," to which we attached a small salary. At first he protested about the salary, but really it thrilled him—it made him a member of "the staff." He would talk about how much he loved all of us and how grateful he was until it was positively embarrassing. We would tell him that the amount of love he felt for us was about the size of *his* heart. It made no difference—those outpourings could not be stopped, nor could the daily tirades against his parents.

One day I was standing near the kitchen when I heard a small crash. I turned and saw that Brazilian John had dropped and broken one of the coffee mugs. We have dozens of such mugs; breaking one was of no importance whatsoever, but the look of terror on his face was astounding to behold. He was visibly trembling, and his eyes filled with tears. He told me that he knew we wouldn't trust him anymore and we would fire him. I hardly knew what to say—his reaction was so out of proportion to a broken coffee mug. I frantically assured him that we would not take away his job—that his work was impeccable and we needed him. Finally he calmed down enough that we could talk about it, and I asked him why on earth he was so fearful about making such a very small mistake. Apparently when he was a kid, breaking a coffee mug would have resulted in being on the receiving end of a heavy belt buckle. He would buy us another mug, which he would pay for himself, and there was to be no argument about it.

When I looked at Brazilian John I often thought about what an extraordinary young man he was and what a tragedy it was that his parents, out of whatever combination of fear and the culture they lived in, were completely missing out by not having him in their lives. One would be so proud to have such an intelligent, courageous, compassionate young man as one's very own son. But then, I have thought this about many young men.

All this was back before we had anything like the AIDS medications we have now. While Dr. Bellman had given Brazilian John many months of a life that had real quality, his body finally began to fail him and he became very ill. He had contracted a raging pneumonia in a body that had already been damaged by too many past fires. Not that he was in any way giving up, he was as feisty as ever. When I went to visit him at Saint Vincent's, he told me he'd be back with us in no time and he was so, so sorry he was letting us down with the cleaning.

He also told me that his mother and father were planning to come to New York and that he was glad they were coming. I was flabbergasted—he'd said nothing about having any contact with his family. He was probably embarrassed to tell us after all his tirades against them. I suspect he was motivated by feeling that he might not have much time left, and to leave this life without ever seeing his family again did not feel quite right no matter how angry he was. The business of his not having much time left was what we all thought, and what none of us wanted to be true. At Friends we try hard to be even-handed with all our clients, and then sometimes one comes along that just gets to us—Brazilian John was such a one.

I recall very clearly walking into Brazilian John's hospital room one afternoon and being greeted by what looked like a Friends In Deed poster. There was my fellow staff member, John Juska, lying on the bed holding him; Winston, one of our African-American clients, was at the foot of the bed massaging his feet; Aline, a young French-woman volunteer, was sitting next to the bed holding his hand; and Larry, a client/volunteer, was putting cold cloths on his forehead. It all looked a bit like a Benetton ad, which didn't stop me from having a small moment of feeling very proud of our staff, our volunteers, and what we were all accomplishing. Brazilian John may have been very ill and frightened, but he was definitely not alone.

Sometimes I'm optimistic that my abilities and skills have evolved to the point where by some act of grace I have become more or less fit for the work I do. Then something happens that makes me feel that I am totally unfit, that I shouldn't be let near a hospital room or a suffering human being. One of those times occurred on another visit to Brazilian John. It was a few days later, and his condition had deteriorated. He was alone in the room, hooked up to oxygen, incoherent, and wild eyed. They had put restraints on his arms for the obvious reason that he was trying to tear out his oxygen tube. He'd clearly taken a real turn for the worse. I went out to the desk and talked to the head nurse, who was not encouraging. Then I called the office and told them to try to find someone who spoke Portuguese who could call the family in Brazil and tell them to come as quickly as possible. I thought next week might be too late.

When I got back to the room, Brazilian John's thrashing was even wilder, and he was pounding his head on the pillow trying to dislodge the damn oxygen tube. I did everything I could think of to quiet him, but he was having none of it. I found myself becoming more frustrated by the minute—it seemed to me that he was making everything so much worse for himself. *Goddammit, Brazilian John—hold still!* I was feeling so angry with him I could easily have smacked him—all my fine compassion out the window. I couldn't get out of that room fast enough.

I was mystified by my behavior. Was I just off balance because I knew he was dying and I couldn't bear it? Or, much worse, did I take it personally if I wasn't successful with my fabulous Mother Teresa–like soothings? Some of both? How could I get into such a fury with a client I cared so much about (or indeed with any client)? I'd never had such a reaction before, and it truly worried me. I have no answers for that day—it's not something that's ever happened again.

Back to Saint Vincent's the next day—afraid of what I might find. What I found was two very small elderly people sitting by the bed, looking at their sleeping son. A pair of little gray mouse-people, confused and sad. The father immediately jumped up and shook my hand, bending forward in a formal little bow, smiling sweetly. We couldn't speak to each other—both his English and my Portuguese being nonexistent. He also could not speak to his son, or rather, he could speak to him but there would be no response. They had arrived too late for that. I made a mental note to ask the Portuguese translator to tell them that we were sure João knew they were there and that he was happy they had come—that we all were.

Brazilian John had fallen into a coma from which I guessed he would leave us. All that fierce struggle, and now he was completely still and peaceful in the bed—partly because he was becoming weaker by the hour, partly because they had given him sedatives to temper his wild ravings and ease the pain. I used my awkward miming skills to encourage his mother and father to talk to him even though their son couldn't respond. Imagine coming all the way from Brazil and arriving in overwhelming New York City, only to find that you are too late and your son is dying. I couldn't even imagine what that must've been like for them.

I looked at the tiny little gray-haired man sitting there and thought about how terrified his son had been of him all his life. It seemed impossible. I looked at the frail little woman, with the saddest face one could ever see. Looking at her, I knew that she may have been too frightened herself to protect Brazilian John when he was a little boy, but that didn't mean she didn't love her son. She loved him very much—it was all over her face. They both looked dazed and heart-broken.

When I stepped off the elevator just outside Brazilian John's room the next day, I immediately came upon his parents in the hallway, huddled together and tearful. Their son had died just a few minutes before. I went into the room to kiss Brazilian John and say good-bye, to tell him how much he meant to us, to thank him. His parents stared at me—I wondered what on earth they made of it all. After a while the translator arrived to help them with the hospital business that needed to be attended to, and through him I communicated my sorrow, told his parents how much we all loved their son and what an amazing and gallant young man he was. As the translator spoke, they stared hard at my face. Surely they must have wondered how it was that this WASP Americana seemed to have such a strong connection to their Brazilian boy. There wasn't really any way to explain it to them, nor was it really necessary, but I could certainly tell them that we would never forget their son.

We have not forgotten Brazilian John; we think and talk about him often. When I got back to Friends In Deed that sad day, I found a very subdued staff—this was one of the more difficult losses we'd experienced over the years. We agreed that there was something rather off about Brazilian John's death—we all felt it—the rather ordinary quiet manner in which he slipped away. He was such a fire-cracker in life—shooting off in every direction—all energy and crackle. We had not expected his death to look like that—going into a coma, then just quietly leaving. We thought he would fly out of his body, whooping and hollering for joy, just like he flew down the streets on his shiny black Rollerblades.

People come and go. There are clients who arrived in our very first year and still come to the Big Groups, though they are now strong and healthy with the new medications. Their health is not the issue anymore, but life keeps happening and they think of Friends In Deed as the place where they can count on support around whatever it is they are having a tough time with. We hear all the time that people begin to feel safe the minute they walk in the door—exactly what we'd hoped for.

If someone arrives initially in a state of terror over a new AIDS diagnosis and then they're in the same room a few years later dealing with the fact that their landlord has just threatened them with eviction, the ensuing dialogue can be very reassuring to newcomers. If all you can think about is dying, if you're sure that your own death is lurking just in the next room, seeing the possibility that one day your biggest worry could be whether or not you might lose your apartment creates real possibility for frightened people who have no vision of a future.

So many of those who were there in the early years are now gone. There are those who have died and those who, because they are no longer in crisis, have simply drifted away. There are also those who never come back after their first Big Group—they tend to be the ones who were hoping for a place where people would commiserate and feel sorry for them. For those people, we are the wrong place. We do not disrespect people by feeling sorry for them. Compassion, yes. Pity, no.

There have been thousands of people. I can't remember them all. Sometimes it's a face I remember and sometimes it's a name but I just can't put the two together. There are those I can't remember and those I can't forget.

CHAPTER 8

Owen was a very intense, tightly wound young man. He came to the Big Groups every week for many years. Each time he walked in the door, he was visibly more fragile, more ravaged by the HIV virus than the time before, yet he steadfastly refused to consider going on any medications. He always raised his hand and went into his lecture about how toxic the medications were and how if you put those things in your body, they might very well kill you. Meanwhile, the AIDS virus *was* killing him. He was putting all his faith in holistic alternatives: acupuncture, supplements and herbs, meditation, et cetera. All very good and valuable things but, clearly, by themselves, they were not extending his life.

There were a couple of things I could say to Owen, some basic principles. I could remind him of the pitfalls that come with our attachment to anything, to any mind-set—how whenever we become adamant regarding a specific position, we narrow our world, we deprive ourselves of possibilities and choices—that the name of the game is always to stay open and flexible. I could remind him that the hundreds of HIV-positive clients at Friends In Deed who were doing so well healthwise were, for the most part, using both Eastern and Western, both holistic and allopathic, medicine—they were taking the medications prescribed by their doctors, and they were also doing everything possible to counteract the toxicity—all those same alternative modalities he believed in. We were simply suggesting that he might think about doing both. I would also point out that something about his choice must be bothering him because otherwise he wouldn't bring it up every time he came to a Big Group.

Whatever I said seemed to roll right off him, and I was always left with having to remind myself that there is a basic Friends principle that *I* must not forget: Each human being has the absolute right to make their own decisions regarding their physical bodies and what they want to put into those bodies—it is no one's business but theirs. Further, it is our job to support people in whatever those choices are no matter how difficult that might be for us. So, frustrating though it was, that's what I did with Owen. One always sensed that he was really terrified but he'd gotten himself wedded to a "position"—he had so labeled himself as a person who didn't take medications that anything else was a threat to his very identity.

There was one other aspect to these exchanges with Owen. I was fully aware that there were many other people in the room who were already on the meds, or about to start taking them, and were also concerned about the toxicity and the side effects. Listening to someone like Owen could really ramp up their fears, and I didn't like to see that happen.

One morning, during the time that we were so concerned about Owen, Robert Levithan called to tell me about Michael, a very dear friend of ours who lived in California; Michael was dying of AIDS, and he wouldn't take any medications either. Like Owen—too toxic.

Robert had just talked to Brenda, Michael's mother, who told him that Michael wasn't doing well, and Robert had decided to fly out to LA the next day. I told him I was planning to go out there in a couple of weeks; he said it didn't sound to him as though we had that much time.

Oh.

I'd go with him the next day.

The combination of Friday the thirteenth and Rosh Hashanah produced a plane flight that was almost empty, a pick-any-seat-you-want sort of flight. Robert was sitting next to me as we flew off to Los Angeles, to the City of Angels, to see the Freiberg family—angels all:

Brenda the mother, Tom the father, Katie the sister, and our darling friend Michael, the beautiful young son who was dying of AIDS. His older brother, Brett, had died of AIDS five years before.

Robert and I had frequent conversations with the family, so we already knew that Michael had AIDS-related dementia. Brenda told us about his going up to strangers on the street and telling them that at one time he had AIDS but that now he was completely cured. In one phone conversation I had with Michael, he told me he was going to move to Rome and he thought I should move there too. Also, he was putting together a show of Native American Huichol art, which he would take all over the world— all the kinds of exciting plans Michael might have been making if he wasn't so weak that he couldn't even sit up in bed without help.

It wasn't only the prospect of seeing Michael that made us heavy of heart, it was also the prospect of looking into the faces of his mother and father—that was the most difficult part for me. They were losing their son whom they loved more than anything in the world, and they had accepted with absolute grace Michael's rejection of allopathic medicine. He would not take the antivirals. He felt a strong connection of the heart to all things Native American and had found a shamanic healer with whom he had spent a great deal of time—certain that this man would heal him—lots of rattles and drums and chanting. Brenda had said to me many times that they honored his choices—that it was his path and he had to do what felt right to him.

Could I do it? Could I be so courageous and wise if it were Max or Fitz? I know it's the right and loving thing to do, and I would wish to do it—but I don't know that I could. In my mind's eye I have an ugly picture of myself screaming with fear, trying to force medications down my son's throat.

I tried to read a little, gazed into space, looked at the gorgeous cottony white clouds that lay below us. It was appropriate that I was making that trip with Robert—in our different ways we had been on the AIDS journey together for a long time, and we were old hands at doing this—this heading toward a room in which someone we loved was dying. We shared a lot of history, too. We met at the Louise Hay workshop where I met Archie. I always remember seeing Robert the first time—blond, handsome, dressed all in white. He was dressed all in white sitting next to me on the plane—Robert loves white, he's famous for it—no one ever gives Robert a gift that isn't white. When we met he was already involved with the Healing Circle, so I would see him there, and that progressed to visiting hospitals together and dinners and movies and then becoming very good friends. In '88 Robert and I joined a spiritual retreat in Santa Fe. We both fell in love with the high desert, and as a result he ended up moving to Santa Fe for a few years. That's where he met Michael who was working in an art gallery there. It's also where I met Michael on one of my visits. Robert's a therapist, so after we opened Friends In Deed he knew he wanted to be part of it and came back to New York—a good thing all around. So we've shared a lot—and now we were on a plane making this sad trip together.

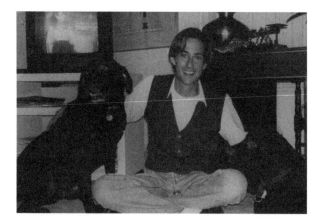

I kept picturing all the times Michael came to New York on art business and stayed with Patrick and me. Many a night, when I dragged myself upstairs at some obscene hour of the early morning, I left Patrick and Michael sitting side by side on the great huge sofa, watching the late, late, *late* movie—each with a cat draped over them. It didn't seem so very long ago.

We arrived at the Freibergs' house in Brentwood, went through the initial greetings, then walked the white-carpeted hall back to the bedroom to see Michael. He was ensconced in Brenda and Tom's big light-filled corner bedroom, with photographs and flowers everywhere, three dogs lying on the floor, and also some familiar-looking grim medical hardware. Michael was propped up on pillows, half dozing, partly medication induced. Brenda said, "Michael, Robert and Cy are here!" His eyes opened and his face lit up when he saw us. The look of him was altered but not profoundly so—he was not emaciated, his color was good.

There were home-care nurses in attendance, on round-the-clock eight-hour shifts. There was constant movement around Michael to keep him as comfortable as possible; comfort was the name of the game at that point. Several times an hour they inserted a tube down his throat to suction his lungs, which were filling with liquid. There was a limit to how much good they could do with the suctioning— the terrible truth was that he was drowning.

There was so much happening, so many people everywhere, so much food everywhere, so much coming and going, that the real trick was to find a space in which to be with Michael for a quiet moment alone. Both Robert and I wanted that badly, and finally, with Brenda and Tom's help, we got it.

In our time together Michael told me he was going to move back to New York tomorrow, wished he'd done it long ago, but he was going to do it now, and we were going to have a wonderful time there. "We can go look at art all the time!" "Oh, how lovely," I'd said. "I can't wait!"

The next day Michael seemed to have a bit more strength, enough that he was carried outside, where he lay on a chaise on their pretty shaded brick patio, beneath a big sheltering tree, surrounded by flowers and insects and birds, the three dogs and several friends and family members who took turns sitting close to him, touching him, talking to him, making plans.

At one moment he said to us loudly and clearly, "I am *not* dying!"

He wanted all of us to go to Orso, his favorite restaurant. When we explained that the restaurant wouldn't be open for a couple of hours yet, he said, "Okay, we'll go later, but now we have to start packing because we're all leaving for Tuscany in the morning! We're taking all the dogs!" As he talked we could see his strength ebbing and his lungs filling as his voice got weaker, and he seemed to shrink beneath the blanket. Michael's presence and energy had always taken up a lot of space—now that great bright light was dimming.

As that day came to a close there was a moment when Brenda, Robert, and I were alone with Michael in his bedroom. He was definitely weaker now. He'd used a lot of energy with going outside and all the talking he'd done—not to mention the medications and suctionings. He had dozed off, and Brenda was sitting on the floor next to the bed, holding his hand. She passionately loved Michael—always had. She was smiling up at him, holding hard to the time that was left and also letting him go. The whole story was on her face. Her tears streamed down. Robert and I wept with her. Everything was absolutely silent. She and Tom were the parents I would wish for for every one of our clients.

A small part of me also wished that Owen were standing there, and that I could say to him, *You see—this is what it looks like—this is what the stubborn refusal to take any medications can look like . . . Is this really what you want?*

Fortunately the bigger part of me knew that both Michael and Owen had their own journey in this lifetime, and the idea that something was going wrong was my error in thinking—that it was real arrogance to assume that I knew how things ought to be. I've often noticed that the more I care for someone—and I adored Michael— the more likely I am to slip into the erroneous notion that something is going wrong. I often have to remind myself that I'm not running the show.

The next morning Robert and I went into Michael's bedroom before leaving for the airport. Michael was not very alert. His eyes opened briefly every few seconds—then quickly closed again. I knew that whatever we said then would likely be the last words between us in this lifetime, the last sight I would have of my darling friend.

I left Robert alone in the room with Michael—very aware of how intense it all was for him. Michael had been one of Robert's very closest AIDS buddies. The plan was that they would do it together, they would survive the virus—together. Now it had come to pass that Robert was strong and well—T-cell count climbing with the new medications—and Michael was leaving. Very, very hard for Robert. I often saw his strong handsome face blur, his eyes fill with tears.

Finally it was my time to say good-bye. I told him I'd be back in two weeks. "That's good," Michael said. The rest of our conversation was very simple: "I love you. I love you, too. I love you. I love you, too."

Long embraces with Brenda and Tom, assurances that we would be in constant touch—out the door.

Late evening two days later, I got home after work, and as I fed the cats I listened to the messages on my answering machine. It was Brenda's voice asking me to call her. I would, of course—but I already knew what she would say.

I remember that I canceled the dinner plans I had for that evening—I didn't feel like talking—certainly not to anyone who didn't know Michael. I thought about how sad Patrick would have been—he hadn't spent as much time with Michael as I had but he'd spent enough to know that Michael was extraordinary, to love their late-night movie sessions, and certainly he, too, would have felt a real personal loss.

I spent that evening lying on the sofa staring into space and petting the cat that was lying on top of me. Like all the other losses I'd experienced in the last couple of years, Michael's death triggered thoughts about my husband's death and the weeks of his dying in the hospital. It hadn't been that long ago. As I lay there, a memory from long before floated to the surface.

✦　✦　✦

Memory: Patrick and I were standing in Max's bedroom watching him in his crib. Our boy was holding on to the crib rail and bouncing up and down. As a baby Max was a great bouncer. When I first went into the room that morning I found he'd bounced his crib clear across the hardwood floor to the opposite wall.

Patrick started singing, "Yes sir, that's my baby! No sir, I don't mean maybe!" I joined in. Max laughed and bounced up and down in perfect rhythm. I assumed he was laughing because he was happy—surely he was too young to be laughing at the fact that neither Patrick nor I could sing worth a damn. Patrick started doing a zany loose-kneed dance all around the room.

CHAPTER 9

On a pleasant fall day in 1963, Patrick went out for a walk, came home, and said, "It's very strange—the construction of Lincoln Center is nearly complete, thousands of people will be there every night, and I don't see any new restaurants being built anywhere in the neighborhood." We looked at each other and said, "My god, wouldn't it be fun?!" Patrick's younger brother, Mike, was now living in New York, having recently gotten out of the service, where he had run the officer's club, liked that job, and was now working for Restaurant Associates to learn and get more experience. Immediately the three of us began fantasizing about having a perfect little place right in the new cultural heart of the city. A couple of days later Patrick took another walk. This time he came back and reported that just across the street from Lincoln Center, down the block on Sixty-fourth Street between Broadway and Central Park West, there was a cement garage for rent. The monthly rent was $465. I have an extremely poor memory for the cost of things; I don't even remember what we paid for the brownstone we bought four years later, but I will never forget that number—now it seems absolutely astonishing—now one might be able to rent a broom closet for that amount. If it were a very small broom closet—maybe.

We talked to brother Mike some more and decided to risk it. All wisdom dictated that we were crazy, everyone was advising against it. We were told over and over again that the restaurant business was impossibly difficult, look how many restaurants opened and closed all the time, we had no experience, we didn't know what we were doing, and on and on. Fortunately we didn't listen. *Three* people with moxie.

We signed the lease and quickly hired a small construction crew with whom we made it all up as we went along—the whole thing was completely ad hoc. For example, one day Patrick was riding along Park Avenue and saw that they were dismantling the old Dobbs hat store, carrying out a lot of beautiful oak paneling, and throwing it into a Dumpster. He stopped the cab, got out, bought the paneling on the spot at a ridiculously low price, and that beautiful age-mellowed wood soon became the old Irish pub bar that it is to this day. That was the spirit of the entire endeavor—it was all more or less a restaurant version of Mickey and Judy looking at the barn and saying, "Hey, this is great—we can do the show right here!"

While we were creating the physical place, Mike decided that if he was actually going to run a restaurant in New York City, it might be a good idea if he learned something about really good food and the preparation thereof (Mike was originally from the part of the country that throws the green beans in a pot with a piece of fatback in the morning then lets them cook all day), so he enrolled in Dione Lucas's cooking school. Dione Lucas was the Julia Child of that time. She had cofounded the Cordon Bleu cooking school in London, she had a cooking school here in New York, she wrote cookbooks, and she taught on television. As great good fortune would have it, when Mike told Dione what we were doing and why he was in the class, she confessed that she was having a very difficult time with the school. She said that she was a terrible businesswoman and didn't really care about being a good one, she was tired of all that, and what she'd love more than anything in the world would be to close the school and go back to her first love—being the chef in a small restaurant. So in a matter of weeks Dione had closed her business and thrown in her lot with us, with the result that soon after we opened we got a rave four-star review from Craig Claiborne, the restaurant critic of the *New York Times*. That original restaurant had only about sixty seats. Thanks to Dione and Mr. Claiborne, all of them were filled all of the time.

The name The Ginger Man came about because while we were

creating the restaurant, Patrick was also in rehearsal for J. P. Donleavy's play of the same name. There had already been a London production with Richard Harris playing the title role, and now Patrick was The Ginger Man. As the look of the restaurant was certainly a direct descendent of the classic Irish pub, the name seemed a natural. Also we liked the provocative quality of it—no one seemed to be quite sure what a "Ginger Man" was. I went downtown to watch a rehearsal the day that Donleavy himself was coming for the first time. He had just arrived from the island where he lived off the coast of Ireland, and everyone was in a lather of excitement and fear—

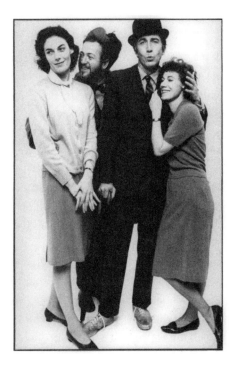

what would the great writer think of the production? At one point Patrick asked him what the title actually meant. Those of us sitting with Donleavy in the audience turned toward him in anticipation, the actors froze in their places onstage, we held our breaths and waited for his answer. And waited. And waited. Then finally it came: "I don't know."

People ask each other where they were when President Kennedy was shot—one of those history-changing moments that inspires the question. I remember exactly where I was. I was at home in our nineteenth-floor Riverside Drive apartment, brilliant afternoon sun was pouring in through the windows, and all was very well with our world. I was in the living room doing I don't remember what. Our housekeeper, Loretta, was out in the kitchen with the radio on low volume. Patrick was still in bed though it was already early afternoon—*The Ginger Man* had opened the night before, and he was exhausted. The play had gotten very good reviews, and we were sure there would be a nice long run. I was knocked out by Patrick's performance in a role that used all his wonderful craziness, and I was feeling happy and proud of him. At that instant my world felt both safe and exciting—that perfect combination.

Then, suddenly, I heard a scream, and Loretta came tearing in from the kitchen, threw herself full-length down on the living room floor, and started beating her fists on the rug, all the while wailing, "They shot him! They shot him!"

It took me several seconds to understand what she was talking about. When I did, I had an instant of thinking her reaction was the appropriate one and wishing I had what it takes to behave in exactly the same way. Lying on the floor screaming was just the thing to do.

I remember walking toward the bedroom, dreading giving the news to Patrick. We didn't know yet whether or not there was a chance the president might survive—so there was a short time lapse before the absolute heartbreak and grief.

The decision was made to close Patrick's play for the rest of that week. We had dinner that night at the Plaza Hotel with eight or ten friends. I don't remember ever choosing the Plaza Hotel for dinner any other time, but that night we all felt pulled to be someplace solid and historical—old New York—for whatever illusion of safety there was within those thick old walls. Our communal sense of loss was devastating.

The play reopened but despite the good reviews, the public was not in much of a theatergoing mood. The houses were small as they were everywhere, and eventually they had to close. So the play *The Ginger Man* ended, but the restaurant The Ginger Man sailed on. The construction was completed; we had a big smashing opening party; we were on our way.

Since none of us had ever been in the restaurant business before, the early days had a kind of Keystone Kops quality—racing to the market to buy things we'd run out of; turning around and discovering that a painting was missing from the wall because we didn't yet know you had to bolt everything down; finding that Dione had only made eight servings of that night's special, which were sold out in the first twelve minutes; looking up and seeing the maître d' turn away an elderly, gray-haired, paint-spattered gentleman because there wasn't a seat to be had, recognizing that it was Marc Chagall who was in the middle of painting the Opera House murals across the street, running after him, escorting him back, and giving him our table. It felt as though we were always just one step ahead of a calamity, but oh my god, it was fun!

Excited as we were then, we really had no idea what was ahead. We never imagined that we would host so many theater parties, openings, and closings, that we would give the New York Film Festival party every year, that while many other restaurants have opened (and many have closed) in the area, that little restaurant we started with not a clue about what we were doing is the one that became forever connected in so many people's minds with Lincoln Center—a New York City icon.

It was brilliant of Patrick to see the possibilities—it was a surprisingly long time before there were any other new restaurants in the area, so we were definitely the place to be. People tell me all the time they can still remember what a big deal it was to be able to get a reservation at The Ginger Man. New Yorkers came before and after performances across the street, and the artists who were in the performances came as well. There they all were, at different tables—George Balanchine, Leonard Bernstein, Andy Warhol, Placido Domingo, Jerome Robbins, and on and on. As a child I don't remember ever hearing politicians or scientists or academicians spoken of with any particular reverence in our family—it was artists that seemed to be admired above all others by both my mother and father. I wasn't given books about Washington and Lincoln, I was given biographies of Bach and Rembrandt. Now there we were with this little restaurant we'd created that was continually visited by many of the greatest artists of our time. And it continues. It absolutely thrilled me then; it still makes me happy.

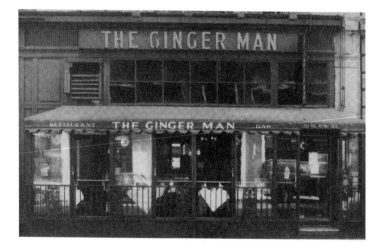

Several years ago the restaurant was renamed O'Neals'; there have been expansions, and the restaurant now seats a couple of hundred people. It's a very good example of what can sometimes happen when you just charge ahead and do something for which you are completely ill equipped and ill prepared, but for which you have great enthusiasm and passion.

Those early Ginger Man days were a golden time in our lives. I can remember many nights when Patrick and I would sit at the bar drinking champagne and eating Dione's fantastic cheeseburgers, which she made with buttery garlicky French bread and perfect mozzarella. We'd sit there for a long time talking and looking around at the small miracle we'd created, feeling that this was how our lives would always be—one wonderful new excitement after another. Given that we sat there sipping champagne through the evening, having a perfectly lovely time, I can see that Patrick's alcoholism hadn't fully kicked in yet—which certainly contributed to how golden that time was.

CHAPTER 10

Longevity is the driving force in Western medicine, and it was extremely difficult for doctors and nurses who were working with AIDS patients during those years when science had almost nothing to offer. The first medication that appeared was AZT, a drug that had crushing side effects for many and didn't really do much other than slow down the progress of the virus somewhat in some people. It definitely did not save lives. If you were in the medical profession and believed that keeping someone alive (no matter what their quality of life might be) was "success" and that dying was "failure," you were going to have a very tough time with a disease like the HIV virus because there was quite a long period when we did not think there were going to be any survivors. There was a lot of talk in those days about burnout, and, of course, there would be if you think that with every death you have failed. How many failures can one doctor or nurse withstand?

The more I came to believe that our physical body is not *who* we are—the lesson I learned from every spiritual teacher I ever came in contact with, the lesson I learned from Archie, the lesson I learned at the Healing Circle—the more comfortable it was for me to sit next to the bed of someone who was dying. It's a perception that is shared by everyone else on the staff of Friends In Deed, as well. We do not experience burnout because we don't think that anything is going wrong, which does not mean that we are not often very, very sad and that we don't feel great compassion for the people who are ill and for the people who love them. However, our sense of loss does not bring with it the frantic quality that comes with thinking that something tragic is happening. We do not bring fear of death into the room with us. Very often the fear that families and friends bring into a hospital room only intensifies the fear of the person lying on the bed. It's completely understandable, and it's sometimes very painful to watch.

I remember in the winter of '91, soon after FID opened, going to visit Marty, one of our clients, in the AIDS ward at Saint Vincent's. His parents had come from their home in the Midwest to visit their very ill son, and Marty had asked me please to be there when they arrived—he was very anxious about their visit. He hadn't seen either his mother or his father in a very long time, and they had been no part of his New York life.

I sat on a folding chair against the wall, watching his father sitting across the room on one of the two padded chairs. From the look of him he clearly would rather have been anywhere else on the planet. He'd said almost nothing from the moment he walked in. Every few seconds he would glance out the window that looked west toward New Jersey. I kept thinking that he probably wished he had wings so he could fly right out that window, though he didn't really look like a man who would entertain such a fanciful notion—but then, you never know. The other thing he did was chew peanuts, which he put into his mouth very methodically, one at a time. He took them carefully out of a little cellophane bag, which made a crinkling sound every time he reached into it. He chewed each peanut for such a long time it seemed impossible there were any peanuts left to chew. It was incredibly irritating. I am a person of many fanciful notions, and the one I had right then was that I would just hurl myself across the room and strangle him.

The other padded chair in that room was for Marty's mother, but all during the time I was there, she never sat in it. She stood right next to the bed leaning over her son, driving him mad. I sat there wondering, *Doesn't she see it? Why doesn't she shut up?* She was telling him all about his sister's garden back home, flower by flower, and how great it was going to be when he made his summer visit for the big barbecue. He would be so proud of his sister, and just wait till he saw the tiny pink sweater she knit for little Lynette—it was just the most cunning thing! Why, there would be so many things to show him next summer! When he came home.

I understood why Marty had begged me to stay with him, but I think his parents very much wondered why I was there—they kept giving me quick sharp little glances.

Marty was the color of old candle wax. He had serious PCP pneumonia—so serious that if the antibiotics he was on didn't improve things by the next day, if he wasn't able to get more air into his lungs, they would have to intubate him. He was terrified of that possibility. I would have been, too. The doctors were also concerned that something might not be right with his liver—the AZT may have done some serious damage. As his mother prattled on and on about all they would do next summer, I figured that the chances of Marty's being alive next summer were right there with my being asked to sing "Mimi" at the Met.

Finally, after I spent about an hour watching this distressing scene, Marty fell asleep, and his mother had to stop talking. Well, I don't suppose she *had* to—but thankfully, she did. The room went silent, and I made my departure.

As I left, walking down that hallway I knew so well, I thought how very, very sad it was that his father could not even speak to his son. I so wished he could break out of the frozen shell he was encased in and tell Marty he loved him and that it was all right and he was there for him. That's all Marty really needed to hear. I also wanted his mother to be quiet and simply say "I love you" instead of all those words that meant nothing—that brought no comfort. But, while I was wishing they could have done what I thought was "right," I reminded myself that in reality they were simply terrified and had no tools to deal with their fear and helplessness. What I had just witnessed was the very best those two people could do, and who the hell was I to think something was going wrong just because I, in my fine enlightenment, thought they should do it all differently? In my ongoing desire to become less judgmental (the most difficult thing in the world for me), more compassionate and loving—some of my toughest challenges are certain parents. Well, along with people who scream into their cell phones on the elevator I'm in.

The fact that I've reached a place where I can actually encourage another human being to leave this life if that's what they need to do has been a long and intense journey. In my former life I most certainly thought that dying was the most terrible thing that could happen unless you were 102 and died in your sleep—if it was someone I knew, I had to do everything I could to prevent it. I always felt to some degree responsible for anyone anywhere in the world around me—including the clerk at the hardware store—I always wondered if there weren't something I could have said or done to save them.

In this regard I went through absolute agony when John Lennon was murdered. I don't mean just the crushing sadness of the loss, I shared that with millions, I mean that I was absolutely caught in the idea that it was in part my fault. I probably would have felt some sense of responsibility given that we lived in the same city, so it was truly excruciating because we lived in the same building.

If you do any renovation of your house or apartment in New York City, the one thing you can absolutely count on is that it will not be finished the day you have to move in—no matter how brilliantly you planned, no matter what promises were made. When we finally had to move into our new apartment in the Dakota, it was a lucky thing that we liked all the workmen because we were going to be together for some time to come. But before that day, in the spirit of trying to move things along as quickly as possible, each morning I would make my way—first through the icy cold streets, then through the wrought-iron gates and the mahogany and marble of the Dakota's public spaces— to check on the progress of the work that was meant to have been finished two months before. While I was there at the construction site, I would smile, frown, cajole, threaten, applaud, and weep.

One morning, when I was leaving our almost-home after checking the progress, I rang for the elevator; as it took a very long time to reach the eighth floor, given the water-and-weights system that runs those elevators, I wandered over to the window and looked out into the courtyard while I waited. It was snowing hard, great fat flakes slowly floating down, and through that lovely veil I could see into the apartments across the way. One window particularly drew me—the window into a big white kitchen where I could see a table in the middle of the room and a man sitting there with a white coffee cup and an open newspaper. There was something invitingly warm and beautifully calm about the scene—I stood there mesmerized. Then, just as the elevator arrived, I realized that the man I was looking at was John Lennon. John Lennon, our hero—the face I followed every moment it was on the screen—the voice I could always pick out from the other three. I was absolutely frozen in place, as if I'd come upon something completely unexpected and surprising, which made no sense because of course I knew he lived in the Dakota—the whole world knew John Lennon lived in the Dakota—it was one of my great excitements about moving into that building. Maybe it was the intimacy of watching him drinking his morning coffee and reading the newspaper in the early light. Whatever it was, I couldn't move. The elevator came, and the elevator went.

Finally the day arrived when it could be said that we were "living" in the Dakota. At last we had a home that was not filled with carpenters and painters, with lumber, paint cans, and sawdust. The results of the renovation were all we had hoped, though it had certainly been frustrating and exhausting to be living in the middle of it for the last month of the work. I made a lot of bad jokes asking the workmen what they would like for breakfast on Christmas morning, since obviously they'd still be there. The animals fared the worst. The day we moved them in, four parakeets were so terrified by the construction noises that they fell right off their perches and we found them lying on their backs with their little twig legs to heaven; one of our cats got herself tiled into a wall for several hours; the dog looked miserable.

Once we'd settled in I created a routine for myself: I had recently been asked to design the costumes for an off-Broadway play, followed by the costumes for a new Paul Taylor dance, which had led me to think that designing costumes was going to be my new life. Now, of course, I could perfectly well have done the drawings and all at home, but if there is anything more romantic than having a "studio," I can't imagine what it is. I loved saying, "Well, why don't you call me later at the 'studio'?" So now, each working morning, I'd get Max and Fitz off to school, then I'd walk the seventy-five blocks down to SoHo to my new space on Wooster Street. Always, as I left our apartment and waited for the elevator, I'd look out the window and almost always, there was John Lennon reading the paper and drinking his coffee. *Good morning, John.*

I really did have to laugh at myself. It's not as though I didn't know I was ridiculous. There were days when I took the elevator closer to the kitchen door, which was the one the Lennons used, and on the way down we sometimes stopped on the seventh floor, and John would get in. He'd say hello. I'd say hello in a voice gone embarrassingly high and squeaky. This happened several times. His physical presence was so powerful I could barely speak. What was it? The year we lived in London, I had many neighborly chats over the fence with Sir Laurence Olivier. I did Elvis Presley's screen test with him. I'd had lunch with Picasso, easy! But with John Lennon I turned to jelly. I had romantic dreams about John Lennon in the dark of the night. I was a complete fool as regards John Lennon.

Early in the evening of December 8, 1980, I was lying on my bed reading until it was time to begin talking my sons into going to bed; Patrick was in LA finishing up a television movie he'd been filming for the past couple of weeks.

I could hear the boys' voices from down the hall as they yelled to each other from room to room—Fitz came in to ask me something about his homework and then, as he headed back, I could hear that he and Max were starting to argue about something—I hoped I wouldn't have to get up, the book I was reading was hard to put down.

Suddenly, at the edge of my consciousness, outside my book concentration, I heard some sharp cracking sounds. In a minute Max appeared at my door and said, "Mom, did you hear that—those were gunshots!"

"Don't be silly! Of course those weren't gunshots!" Max ran back to his room, and I went back to my book.

A few minutes later Max was in the doorway again.

"John Lennon's been shot . . . I heard it on the radio."

No.

I tried to buy a few seconds by getting annoyed with Max, telling him that it was a very poor joke. But of course I knew—the way you know. I jumped off the bed; I thought about racing down the stairs but I was too frightened of what I might find to do that. We turned on the television and watched the horror unfold, terrible detail by terrible detail. As with Kennedy, I had the desperate prayerful hope that somehow he was superhuman, that he would survive even such massive damage. There wasn't the waiting time there was with the president—it was almost immediate that we knew we had lost him. We watched the camera follow Yoko Ono as she left the hospital.

The phone rang—Patrick in a voice gone all tight and gravelly told me that he'd be able to finish and come home the next day—he'd get the earliest possible plane. He wanted to know if I was all right. Neither of us was all right.

Two things began almost immediately—hundreds of voices from the street below—"All we are saying is give peace a chance"—and the voice in my head saying that I somehow should have saved him.

How could I not have saved him when I loved him so much?

Sleep was impossible. Hundreds and hundreds of voices chanting the mantra "All we are saying . . ." I was glad all those people were down there—it meant I wasn't alone. I kept thinking about the apartment across the courtyard and what it must be like within those walls. I kept thinking I should have saved him.

I did not sleep that terrible night.

The next morning I was exhausted. The voices from below didn't stop and neither did the ringing of my telephone. All our friends were calling: Was I at home? Did I hear the shots? What was it like at the Dakota? What about Yoko? Had I seen Mark David Chapman?

I had.

I should have known.

No one could get their mind around the horror of what had happened, everyone was driven to talk about it, parse the details over and over—John Lennon meant so much to everyone we knew—like John Kennedy, he was ours. He was us.

At one point I noticed that there was something seductive about the celebrity of being the one who was at the scene, the one with some inside info. I noticed, and it didn't feel good.

Finally I decided I needed a break from talking about it—I needed to go outside, get some air. I decided to do some errands I'd been putting off. When I got to the gates of the building, I was staggered by what I saw. I'd had no idea. During the night the great enormous entrance to the Dakota had become a shrine. The gates and walls were covered with flowers and notes and letters. Candles were burning everywhere. The street was blocked off, filled with thousands of people. Boom boxes were playing—mostly "Imagine." The chanting went on and on: "All we are saying . . ."

I had never seen anything remotely like it in all my life.

The Dakota was completely locked down. I was told that no one would be allowed in unless they lived in the building—no bringing your order from the wine shop, no friend for a playdate with your kid, no delivery of the gown from Bergdorf's you needed to wear to the party that night—nothing.

One fear was that someone from the media would sneak in—the other that when something insane happens, it often attracts more insanity. Leonard Bernstein had already received a note saying that he was next.

A policeman came inside to lead me out. As we walked through the gates I could see that the attention of every single person in that enormous crowd was focused on me. I came from John's building. I was one degree closer to John. I met the eyes of some of the people in front—eyes filled with tears, theirs and mine. As the policeman walked me out, he put a protective arm around me as he maneuvered me through the packed bodies. Both he and I joined the chanting as we inched our way through.

That evening there were a lot of us crowded into the Bernsteins' apartment. It was a very subdued gathering—friends who simply needed to be together in the same room in that sad terrible time. We were all ragged from lack of sleep, and we didn't quite know what to do with ourselves—we talked of wandering around, not really being able to concentrate on anything—but mostly we talked of what John Lennon had meant in our lives and the wonder of how powerful he was in the world. I kept looking at the door, waiting for Patrick to walk in. I'd left word downstairs, telling him where I'd be.

When he arrived, he walked over to me—fast—eyes full of tears. I thanked god I wasn't married to a man who wouldn't cry over the murder of John Lennon.

After four or five days the tone of everything changed. In front of the building, it went from a street filled with people, who were there out of sorrow and love, to a great number who were there because they hoped to get their face on camera—their moment of celebrity. The street was becoming littered with cigarette stubs and beer cans, and the mood was becoming raucous and slightly hostile—at least toward those of us who lived there.

The Dakota staff was exhausted from working round the clock, the tenants were pitching in, helping out with running the elevators, photographing everyone, and making name tags so that we could be recognized immediately and admitted to the building. I spent a few hours each day receiving and recording a part of the mountain of flowers Yoko was having sent on to hospitals, nursing homes, and the like. She had also arranged for food to be sent down to the building staff; she was clearly mindful how hard both they and the police were working—how very tired and stressed they must be. To show such concern and awareness at that moment—how was it possible? I was told she explained to their son, Sean, that his father was killed by a very sad, very sick man and that they must not hate him for what he had done.

I myself did not seem to be exhibiting the same compassionate spirit. I was beginning to feel a real dislike for some of my fellow tenants, the ones who made it clear that they thought what was going on was all a dreadful inconvenience—the ones who didn't seem to have had their hearts broken. I had no tolerance for them at all.

On the fourth day I was bone tired. I thought that the night before might be a night of real sleep. Instead, from the floor above, came the unbroken pounding of drums all night long. When I complained about it the next morning, I was told it was Julian—John's son.

Well, none of it would have happened if only I'd had my wits about me and known when I saw Chapman standing outside the building that he was dangerous. I just couldn't believe I didn't know. There was always a small knot of young fans who were made to stand in a specific area on the sidewalk just to the right of the entrance. Chapman was there for two or three days—tall, blond, slightly overweight, bland of face, with the soft pudgy look of a baby—nothing obviously sinister about him at all, a perfect prototype of those killers whom neighbors later describe as appearing to be completely harmless: *Why, he seemed so nice—he kept to himself mostly, kind of a loner—always very polite— like I said, he seemed to be a perfectly nice fellow.*

I saw him there a few times, smiling and talking with the others. Why didn't I know? I just couldn't believe I didn't know.

A few days after John Lennon's death, there was a memorial gathering in Central Park that included a few minutes of silence. Patrick and I went up to the roof of the Dakota and looked down on the many thousands of people, all standing, blanketing the lawns and the pathways of our park—John and Yoko's park. The day was cold and clear and crisp, and in the silence I could not hear a single sound anywhere in the city—there was only the measured beat of the news choppers overhead—it seemed that this entire great city was mourning John Lennon.

After a time things in the exterior world moved back toward normal as they almost always do. In my interior world, my dreams and my waking thoughts were unendingly inhabited by guilt and regret. Why didn't I get that Chapman was dangerous when I saw him standing there by the gate day after day? Why was my intuition asleep so that I failed to sound the alarm? Why wasn't I walking into the Dakota at an hour when I could so easily have been walking in? Why didn't I see Chapman take out the gun? Why didn't I run and

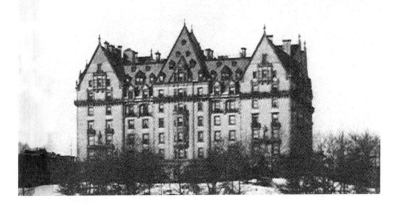

grab his arm, deflecting the bullet? In my grief and obsession I became like a teenager who'd read too many action comics. I knew I was being absurd, but I couldn't stop telling myself that I should have been able to save John Lennon.

CHAPTER 11

After a time clients with AIDS began bringing not only friends who had AIDS but also friends who had cancer to the Big Group. It occurred to them that the support they were getting from Friends In Deed, the principles they were learning and working with, would be just as valuable around any life-threatening illness. They were right, of course, and now we have clients dealing with many serious diagnoses and the majority of those who are not HIV positive are cancer patients. For most people "AIDS" is a frightening word; it's a relatively new addition to the language—it arrived in the early '80s. The word "cancer" has been terrifying people for a very long time—my mother always said the word in a whisper, that's how terrifying she thought it was.

Initially everything about AIDS was new to me. Cancer was well-known territory. My two closest New York women friends had both had cancer.

Our first year in New York together Patrick did a summer-replacement television series called *Diagnosis Unknown*. It was a precursor to all the shows we now have that solve crimes through forensics. Patrick played the head honcho, and one of his lab assistants was Phyllis Newman. Phyllis was married to Adolph Green, who, together with his partner, Betty Comden, had written *Singin' in the Rain*, *On the Town*, *Bells Are Ringing*, et cetera. In short order the Greens and the O'Neals became great friends. At that time Phyllis and Adolph gave a party almost every week, and we met not only actors and directors but all of the Broadway musical theater in their living room: Stephen Sondheim, Jerome Robbins, Bob Fosse, Cy Coleman, Jule Styne—and on and on. Those nights were terrific fun and often

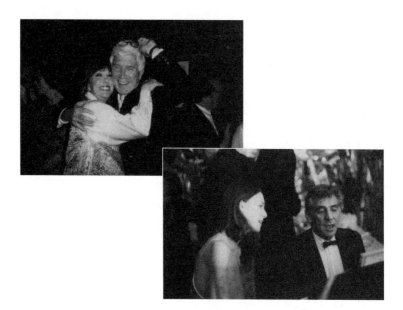

ended around the piano. It was dazzling stuff and a very long way from the San Fernando Valley.

Adolph's best friend was Leonard Bernstein, so soon we were going to the Bernsteins' parties as well, sitting in Lenny's box at his concerts. As time went on, Felicia Montealegre Bernstein also became my close friend—there was a long period when I talked to Phyllis every day and Felicia most days.

Patrick and I arrived at the Greens' one night for a small dinner. Felicia and Lenny were supposed to be there, but they weren't because Felicia had just had a routine mammogram and something did not look good—they were not feeling very sociable. The whole color of the evening changed when we heard the news, but as you do, we all told each other that it would be a false alarm, happens all the time, Felicia would be just fine—anything else was unthinkable.

She eventually was just fine, but not till after she'd had and recovered from a mastectomy. Felicia having cancer was very concerning, but there was just a slight feeling of remove because she was several years older than Phyllis and me. I don't remember it making me any more aware of my own physical vulnerability, my own mortality, than I'd ever been before in my life. Cancer was something that happened to people who were older, and Phyllis and I weren't older.

Then one day, out of the blue, everything changed—did a complete U-turn: Phyllis called to tell me *she'd* had a routine mammogram and that *she* needed a biopsy right away. I was stunned—nothing like this was supposed to happen. Just a few days before, Jerry Robbins had been at one of their parties, and Phyllis and I started dancing for him—we'd most likely had a glass of wine or two—through the rooms, up and down the stairs, and all the while we kept saying to Jerry, "Now don't you dare steal any of this choreography! Don't even think about it!" That was the sort of thing Phyllis and I were meant to be doing—dancing around the room like a pair of loonies for Jerry Robbins—not having biopsies, for god's sake!

As we had with Felicia, we assured each other it was only a technicality and that certainly everything would be absolutely fine. Well, it wasn't fine—not fine at all. A double mastectomy followed, from which Phyllis recovered very well, but it was a shattering experience. More so for her than for me, obviously, but I was frightened too. We still thought of ourselves as very young—this simply was not in the plan. No one in the world was more full of life than Phyllis Newman Green, and now, for the first time ever, Phyllis felt vulnerable and for a period of time did not have her usual sass. Everything in our world shifted.

Felicia's breast cancer and her mastectomy all seemed fairly routine in the world of medicine; she recovered well, there was no evidence of the cancer having metastacized. However, if I thought about it, I was always uneasy about her health because she was a ferocious smoker. Two years after the mastectomy, she and I went to Greece together for a couple of weeks, and as we drove through the mountains of Crete in a tiny little car, I was enveloped in a solid dense gray cloud of cigarette smoke every inch of the way. Even Patrick did not light each new cigarette from the one he was just finishing. The smoke was so all-consuming that I became somewhat anxious about my own health. At one point she said to me, "Oh, I know, sometimes I'm afraid I'm overdoing it." Overdoing it? I would say so.

Then, one night in the spring of '76, I went to the Dakota (we were not living there yet, though very soon we would be) to have dinner with Lenny and Felicia, after which we planned to see Fellini's *Casanova* at a theater just a couple of blocks away. It turned into a particularly jolly evening because after dinner we drifted to the piano and the three of us started singing "Ramona," "Red River Valley," and "Streets of Laredo," old pop Western songs from the '40s. We really threw ourselves into it. The singing was loud and enthusiastic, and Lenny was fortissimo. At that point their younger daughter, Nina, came into the room and stared at us open mouthed. First she couldn't believe that the three of us knew all those lyrics, and second she couldn't understand why we'd want to because she thought they were the silliest songs she'd ever heard. The three of us immediately began trying to convince her that these were great songs by singing more and louder—Nina was not convinced. We were having such a great time that when the moment came to leave for the movie, we didn't really want to. Then we told each other that if we didn't go now, when the film was so nearby, we might never see it, and as we were all great Fellini fans we talked ourselves into it and tore ourselves away from the piano.

It was there, in the semidarkness of the movie-house, that I heard something that froze my blood. We were watching the film, and suddenly Felicia had a fit of coughing. It wasn't that bad, it didn't last all that long, but I heard something. There was a sound to that cough, a sinister sound—and somehow I knew. I thought, *Oh my god, I think we're in trouble here . . . I don't think that pain she's been having in her back is muscular as the doctors have been telling her.* I thought about that trip to Greece and there never being a moment when she didn't have a cigarette in her hand, a cigarette in a short white Aquafilter. Those memories and images sped through my mind as I sat there in the half dark, feeling ill with fear, trying to tell myself I was crazy.

Over the next few days there were doctors' appointments and tests and the beginnings of real concern. Felicia was put in the hospital for some further testing, a bronchoscopy, other unpleasant procedures. Finally the word came. Yes, it was lung cancer—they were going to start a regime of chemotherapy.

I happened to be alone with her in her hospital room when they brought in the apparatus to administer the first IV dose. She was unbelievably light and easy about it all—amazingly brave. When the liquid chemo began to drip into her arm, she hunched up her shoulders, turned her hands into claws, made evil slits of her eyes, and protruded her front teeth in fanglike fashion—a comic horror film monster. That she would turn what was happening into farce was enormously reassuring to me—surely this couldn't be anything terrible if she was making such fun of it.

There was also another quintessential Felicia moment that occurred in her hospital room during that time: She'd had a fair amount of chemo by then and as a result was feeling really rotten; the minute I walked in I could see that she was in very bad shape. I went over to the bed, leaned down, and said, "Oh, my darling Felicia, is there anything in the world that I can do for you?" "Yes," she said. "Never get another perm!"

None of us who were her friends have ever stopped remembering and talking about Felicia Montealegre Bernstein: She was the best, the most beautiful, smartest, wittiest, and to be at her bedside, both in the hospital and at home, watching her die was a heartbreaking experience—certainly the first such experience I'd ever had.

That time with Felicia was when I first learned to just be there and be quiet. It's when I first learned how important it is to support someone who is very ill in doing it their way. The truth was that the way Felicia was doing it made me crazy. I did not like her doctor. I thought he was an arrogant jerk. At one moment I was with Lenny when he asked the doctor how Felicia was doing. The reply was, "She's doing very well; unfortunately, the cancer's doing better." I wouldn't have let that man treat my pet gerbil, but when I suggested she have a consultation with someone else—only that, just a consultation—she wouldn't hear of it. No, no, Dr. H. was her doctor and that was the end of it. When I suggested that it might be a good idea to look into vitamins or supplements that could possibly alleviate some of the effects of the extremely toxic chemo she was on, the answer was much the same: "No, no, the doctor hasn't said anything about vitamins or things like that, and I am completely in his hands." So finally I realized that part of it wasn't any of my business: It was not up to me, and I had to shut up. From that moment on I just agreed with and supported. It was a powerful lesson to learn, and it has stood me in good stead at Friends In Deed. It's fine to make suggestions as long as I don't mind having my brilliant suggestions completely ignored.

That bit of wisdom was just one of the things Felicia left me, along with memories of untold hours spent sitting together in her living room or mine or on the porch in the country, making needlepoint cushions and crocheting afghans and talking and talking. After all these years I still carry many of those funny little moments that stick in the mind that seem completely unmemorable but one never forgets them—like an argument we had because we were given very dry chicken sandwiches and Felicia wouldn't let me go into the kitchen to put more mayonnaise on them because it might upset the housekeeper. She and I were once discussing a woman we both knew slightly, who in our eyes had no particular discernable charm but had had three very attractive husbands. I said, "What do you suppose it is?" Felicia said, "It must be some sort of gripping device!"

One night we were in an Upper West Side apartment, guests at a party being given by a couple who were very much a part of the New

York art scene at the time. Our host took the evening and his role very, very seriously and began conducting the whole evening as though it were a late-nineteenth-century art salon. At one point he introduced an Italian concert pianist and said that now the two of them were going to play some duets for us. Everyone was a bit startled when the concert pianist was given the *segundo* parts and the host himself took the *primo*. As they were playing, Patrick leaned over to me, pointed to a gray shape on the left side of a painting hanging next to the piano, and in a whisper asked me what I thought that shape was meant to represent. In the spirit of the seriousness of this extremely artistic evening, I looked hard at the painting and gave it a lot of thought. Finally I was forced to say, "I don't know." Patrick whispered, "Actually, it's the shadow of the lamp on the piano."

It was the perfect send-up for this slightly pretentious evening, and I began to laugh, which I tried to control because, of course, they were still playing. The host began looking over his shoulder at me with a great frown, which only made me laugh harder until finally I bumped the edge of the table next to me and a glass of red wine spilled all over the gentleman sitting on the other side. The host jumped up and started mopping up his guest, and I, still finding it all pretty funny, said perhaps I'd better go home. I thought I was making a joke. In two seconds our host was working my arms into the sleeves of my coat, and we were out the door. Once we got outside Patrick and I were laughing so hard we were leaning on parked cars. The one other laughing face I'd seen in that room was Felicia's—she clearly loved what was happening—everyone else looked very concerned. The next morning she called me and said, "I've always been quite fond of you, but last night you were magnificent!"

It's a terrible thing to lose a friend like that.

The first non-HIV-positive clients to show up at Friends were women dealing with cancer. Some of them were a real challenge for all of us. They began by wanting us to provide a support group just for women with cancer. We would not do that because one of the fundamental principles at FID is "no categories." We do not divide people up according to their issues. If what we were talking about in the Big Groups were treatments and medications, there might be a reason to separate groups. But we're not. We're talking about the emotions—we're talking about anxiety, depression, hopelessness, fear, and these feelings are the same for everyone regardless of their diagnosis. We offer pragmatic spiritual and emotional support, not medical advice.

One evening there was a woman standing in the doorway to the Big Group looking very doubtful about coming in. She said, "I can't go in there—those are all men with AIDS—they have no idea what it's like to be a woman with breast cancer." She told me she'd just been diagnosed, and when I asked her how she was doing she said she was terrified. I called over a young man who was standing nearby who I knew had recently received an AIDS diagnosis. I asked him how he was feeling about his diagnosis, and he said he too was terrified. I could see on that woman's face that she got the point. She went into the room and sat down.

But there were many who weren't quite that easy. Many of the women in those days seemed to feel a kind of entitlement, a *This should not be happening to* me! attitude. It was a bit hard to take when contrasted to all the men who were so ill—not only did they not feel that anything had gone wrong but, on the contrary, that they deserved this terrible thing that was happening to them and it was only right that they get sick and die. Some of our toughest work at Friends had always been to help those fine valuable young men shift that desperately wrongheaded perception, to make them understand that what was happening was an enormous challenge but most definitely not a punishment. A few women, too, went down the road of feeling they were being punished, but more seemed to feel that they were powerless victims of a wildly unfair mistake. Then there were those who already knew that it was simply "what is," and they wanted to learn how to deal with "what is" in the very best way possible. Certainly we have always had clients who arrive already knowing full well that their lives may be greatly enriched by what they are facing.

Over time, men with cancer began to walk in our door as well—recently prostrate cancer seems to be almost an epidemic. At this point, though it took awhile to get there, all the men and women in the Big Group who are dealing with cancer seem to know that they are definitely in the right place. We now see the same kind of courage and willingness to use what is happening in their lives as an opportunity that we have seen for years in clients infected with the AIDS virus.

There is a phenomenon we've heard of more than once: Someone will contract an illness or be in an accident that is not life threatening, and when they go to the doctor or hospital to be treated, in the process something far more serious is discovered. Sometimes that initial event, which appeared to be a "bad" thing, is what saves their lives.

One night a tall beautiful young woman named Mary Beth arrived at Big Group with one of those stories. She was riding her bicycle through the New York City streets when she was hit by a car. She was taken to the hospital. Among other serious injuries, she had hit her head. When they examined her for concussion, they discovered a brain tumor that proved to be malignant.

We have never seen anyone handle such a potentially frightening diagnosis with more grace and courage than Mary Beth. I sat with her while her brain surgeon showed us numerous photographs of her brain and explained that he could go only so far because the line between cancer tissue and brain tissue was ill defined, and going too far meant the possibility of cutting into the brain itself, which he did not want to do—it also meant that, of necessity, he might have to leave some of the cancer tissue and that following up with radiation was a possibility. I visited her within hours after surgery, and instead of the groggy, half-conscious, wounded creature I expected to find lying on the bed, there she was—sitting up, beautiful head wrapped in gauze, eating and chatting away, as clear and articulate as ever. The only time we ever saw Mary Beth exhibit any real fear was after being told by her doctors that she needed both radiation and chemotherapy. She spoke in the Big Group and was clearly pretty freaked out. "I am so fucking scared!" she said with tears streaming down her face. For her the idea of putting that toxic poisonous stuff in her body was far worse than surgery on her brain. For most people it would have been the reverse.

At such times there is usually an immediate shift on people's faces if you say to them, "Well, then, don't do it." That's what happened that night with Mary Beth. I reminded her that because the doctors thought it was the best thing for her to do didn't mean she had to do it. There have been dozens of people in the Big Groups who have complained about how many meds they have to take and how irritating the whole thing is, not to mention the side effects. All you have to do is suggest they stop taking them, and the whole thing changes. In that moment they realize they actually do want to do what the doctor is advising, they do want to live, and they're afraid not to take their doctors' advice. The situation switches from their being victims to being people who are making their own choices, running their own lives. In some cases they do decide to go against their doctors' orders, but now it's a choice they feel clear about. Mary Beth chose to go ahead with the radiation. I went with her for the first treatment, and at that point she was absolutely courageous about that as well. For whatever combination of reasons—and I suspect her spirit is one of the major ones—Mary Beth is doing beautifully. She has frequent checkups, and the remaining cancer seems to just quietly stay where it is without causing any trouble whatsoever.

There was a lovely young schoolteacher named Mindy who had a particularly rare form of cancer that she'd battled for years, during which there were periods of great physical and emotional suffering. While she had a lot of very good, caring women friends, she was not in a relationship. The boyfriend she had had left (I think her illness probably just wore him out), so now she lived alone, which was very frightening for her—emptiness in the night. She was always at the Big Group except for those times when she was too ill to get there. She always raised her hand. She always spoke. She always thanked us. Mindy was one of those people who sometimes complained, sometimes felt sorry for herself, but underneath it there was an iron courage, and I used to wonder if I could possibly do it so well. She also always sat in the same seat, and though she died several months ago, I still expect to see her there.

There's a marvelous woman named Melissa who weekly enters the room in an explosion of color. She is perfectly capable of wearing lime green trousers, a floating lavender tunic, scarves and beads of many colors around her neck, a floppy orange hat, and brilliant red shoes. Her cancer is now in remission, but when she first arrived there were fear and surgery and all the attendant cancer issues. Then when she was well on the road to recovery, her beloved best friend/ sister died from ALS, and a year and a half later her brother in Florida died of the same disease. At every meeting she attends Melissa raises her hand and tells the hard truth about what is going on in her life and everything she feels about what is going on. When she's assessing her own feelings and behavior, she is both compassionate and relent-lessly tough on herself. Melissa qualifies as a Friends In Deed client in every category: She's had a life-threatening illness herself, she's been a caregiver many times over, and she certainly has dealt with grief and loss. That walking rainbow is as powerful a demonstration of our work as any AIDS client we have ever had.

Having people in the Big Group who are dealing with other life-threatening illnesses is very helpful for the people who are HIV positive. It breaks a sense of "specialness." There are things that *are* special about the HIV virus—the fact that it targeted young gay men before it spread all over the world, the fact that it is most often trans-mitted through sex or IV-drug use with all the ancillary judgment that it brings—but there is nothing "special" about the fear. That's universal.

It feels right and proper to widen our parameters. The cancer epidemic has been around for a very long time and doesn't come with the kind of heightened drama there was in the early days of the AIDS epidemic, but being told you have cancer is still and always a crisis for anyone hearing those words.

CHAPTER 12

When Friends In Deed opened, the O'Neal family was no longer living in the Dakota. In fact we'd been gone for quite a while. The thrill of living in that building was heavily shadowed for me by John Lennon's death, and also Patrick and I both felt a pull to get back downtown where we had begun our life in New York. The Upper West Side had lost a lot of the character it had when we first moved there. Back then, in the early '60s, Columbus Avenue had some grit to it—there were dingy little stores and Irish bars frequented by gentlemen who began their drinking early in the day. Now Columbus Avenue was paved with small high-price boutiques and fancy food stores. It was definitely not the same. I don't think that part of it bothered Patrick so much, but I always get a bit uncomfortable when things get too tidy.

For a couple of years we rented a beautiful little house in SoHo on MacDougal Street, then we went even farther south and bought a two-story loft on Warren Street in TriBeCa, which is where we were living in 1991 when Friends opened. It was a terrific space—big and airy with huge brick fireplace that actually worked (not always the case in New York City), and the renovation from the original factory was so well done that for once we felt no need to do any construction before we moved in. There was an excellent big open kitchen, and I cooked a lot of dinners for our uptown friends for whom coming to us felt like visiting a foreign country—so far away was it from their world. In reality it was about 120 blocks from their world. I thought living there was great. The adventure of leaving what had been our physical world for so long—new market, new dry cleaner, new shoe repair, new everything . . .

✧ ✧ ✧

Memory: When I think about the Twelfth Street apartment, I immediately see the dog on the table. When I think about Warren Street,
I immediately see a cat on a table—also a dinner table—a long one
surrounded by a dozen people. The cat was a big striped tabby we'd
rescued from the ASPCA, and his name was Chopper. For completely mysterious reasons that cat could never abide a lit candle.
That night I'd placed eight candles in a line down the center of the
table. As we all watched, Chopper jumped up, started at one end,
and walked the length of the table, smashing his paw down on each
candle as he got to it. He'd pause between each one and shake the
paw that now had hot wax on it, and then proceed. Twelve adults
stared with open mouths, not saying a word—loud applause at the
end.

✧ ✧ ✧

Patrick being an alcoholic was the source of many a crisis over the
years, but in the post-Dakota years he was in good recovery; he was
sober, going to AA meetings regularly, and hanging out with his pals
in the twelve-step programs—those were years when I was not worried about my husband's drinking and drugging. However, if you're
intent on a life free of upset, you'd best not have any teenage sons—
certainly not in New York City. It was undeniably scary out there
(though from what I read and heard, it was pretty damn scary everywhere). I remember weekend nights when Patrick and I were
watching television and that ubiquitous announcement would appear
on the screen: IT'S TEN O'CLOCK—DO YOU KNOW WHERE YOUR
CHILDREN ARE? We'd look at each other, shrug, and finally just laugh
at the absurdity of the question. We had no real idea where our boys
were. We knew where they *said* they'd be. But, where were they
really? This was before cell phones.

There were more or less minor concerns about the boys on an almost daily basis. Fitz was a classically uncommunicative teenager, so we were often worrying about what was really going on with him; Max was more overt trouble, and there were already indications that he might have his father's disease of addiction. There were a lot of concerning incidents, and then one night, when we were in that MacDougal Street house, there was a real horror show.

It was three in the morning, and Patrick was in Florida at the Pritikin Center where he'd gone for two weeks of diet and exercise—all designed to lengthen his life. I was sound asleep in the top-floor bedroom when something awakened me and I slowly become aware that from below I was hearing the sound of loud angry voices coming up the stairs, pushing through the closed bedroom door. I sat up—the better to hear what was going on—and I quickly knew that something not very good was going on. I grabbed my robe and ran down the stairs, where a horrifying sight greeted me. The front door was wide open, Max was lying on the floor with two guys I'd never seen before on top of him, beating on him. There was blood on his head and face. Fitz, thank god, was on the phone calling the police. I immediately began yelling at the two young men: *"Get out of this house—right now!"*

When they saw me, they jumped up and ran out the door and down the stairs. They passed the cops on the way, paused a moment to tell them that Max had a gun, and then they were gone. I heard a car race off into the night.

Three policemen tore into the house, shouting, *"Where's the gun? Where's the gun?!"* One young cop shoved his face into mine, demanding that I tell him where the gun was. I told him that I didn't know what he was talking about—"We have no guns in this house." Nothing so far had frightened me more than the look on that young policeman's face. He was terrified. The idea of a loose gun had clearly scared him to death. It appeared to me that he was so out of control that any crazy thing could happen.

By now an ambulance had arrived as the frantic search for a gun was taking place (this search failed to find the razor blade taped to a wooden handle, which one of the intruders had dropped on the floor as he ran out—the razor blade with which one of them cut Max's head, the cause of all the bleeding). I saw one of the paramedics standing over Max, who was lying on the floor, and I heard him say, "With the amount of alcohol that's in this kid, we'd better keep him walking!"

They got Max on his feet, walked him around a bit, then seated him in a chair and carried him, chair and all, out to the waiting ambulance. They handcuffed him to a chrome bar on the wall of the ambulance, and drove off to Saint Vincent's to check out his injuries and stitch up his head.

This was tough stuff. I was very frightened. Why in the name of god wasn't Patrick there? I wouldn't even be able to reach him for several hours—the Pritikin Center switchboard did not operate at 3:30 a.m. I knew that I had to get some help, I couldn't do this all by myself. I called my brother-in-law, Mike, who said he'd be right down and meet me at the hospital. I also called David and Danielle, close friends of Patrick and mine. They jumped in a taxi and headed downtown. They were the best possible friends to have around me right then—they knew all about alcohol, the abuse thereof, and the craziness it can bring with it. There would be no judgment, only support.

We all met in the emergency room of Saint Vincent's hospital, where we, along with two policemen, waited for them to attend to Max. My son sitting there, head down, hair matted with blood, was a pretty sad-looking creature. It seemed to me that they were taking their sweet time getting to him—but I guess at such a time I would think that. At last a doctor and a nurse took him into a room along with one of the policemen. Half an hour later he reappeared, a portion of his head shaved, several stitches under the bandage. We headed for the police station.

Standing in that police station, looking at my handsome son—my adored son—with his hands secured behind his back, illuminated by the ghastly glow of the overhead fluorescent light, his face impassive, working hard to appear cool, I knew he had to be frightened but he didn't let it show.

How was this possible? This could not be happening! Our Max?

Max at three, running up onto the beach waving his hand in the air after being knocked down by a wave, yelling, *"Taxi!"*

Max leaning back in his high chair, crossing one chubby little leg over the other, raising his half-eaten apple ceilingward, saying, "My compliments to the tree!"

Max, who, when he was little, followed me everywhere, preferring to have a good grip on some part of my clothing, or his face pushed into my neck.

This same Max, handcuffed, standing in the First Precinct, bathed in ghoulish lighting, trying to appear the cool dude, like this was no big deal.

I thought it was a very big deal.

It took about an hour to do what they do in police stations. A fair amount of paperwork and questioning Max, all of which resulted in our being sent home—no gun was found, there was nothing to charge him with.

When we walked outside we saw that the sun was coming up. Five very exhausted, sad people got into taxis and headed for their respective homes. An hour or so later I reached Patrick. He felt terrible that he wasn't there—he'd come home right away. I persuaded him not to do that—it was all over and done. That particular incident was anyway. I was okay. A bit shaken as the immediate fear drained off, but okay.

CHAPTER 13

Every now and again, most often after a Big Group, someone asks me about my credentials, wants to know what and where my training was. They often seem taken aback when I tell them I have no credentials whatsoever. "I've had a noisy life!" I sometimes say. I have had a noisy life, and what shows up in such a life can teach you more than any classroom.

In a sense my real education began with Patrick's alcoholism. For the first several years of our marriage, my husband appeared to be a good old ordinary social drinker. We'd have dinner, both drink a couple of glasses of wine—end of story. Well, I suppose there was the odd exception—a night of our drinking grasshoppers, of all things, at a bar in Malibu until two in the morning and not being able to move or speak for several hours the next day comes to mind. But generally speaking my husband appeared to be an everyday social drinker. Then, in a stroke, all that changed.

It was 1961. We had left our apartment in the Village and moved to the Upper West Side to an apartment on Riverside Drive. Even before things got really scary, I remember thinking, *This ought to be a wonderful time—I thought this would be a wonderful time—why the hell isn't it?* Patrick was on Broadway, starring in the new Tennessee Williams play *The Night of the Iguana*, and at that time to be in a new Tennessee Williams play was the ultimate actor's dream. Not only that, Tennessee had written the play *for* Patrick. It was first done as an Actors Studio production at the Festival of Two Worlds in Spoleto, Italy. At that point it was a one-act play. Back in New York, people heard about the success of the production, so when we returned, they gave a week of performances at the Actors Studio.

Tennessee flew into town to see it, and after the performance he hurried up to Patrick and said, "Well, baby, I think I'd better make this a full-length play for you!"

I heard it. I was standing right there. My breath stopped and so did Patrick's. The greatest playwright of our time is writing a play *for* him!

So again, why wasn't this a fabulous time in our lives? Maybe because doing that play seemed to fill Patrick with anxiety rather than with joy? Something like that.

Had the new producers decided to present the play with the original cast of all Actors Studio people, things would probably have been very different. Instead, in order to beef up the box office they decided to up the ante with some big names. The biggest mistake was to cast Bette Davis in the third part. Ms. Davis was not comfortable having the third biggest role, and she created nothing but trouble from the get-go. She went so far as to react to the huge applause she got when she made her entrance by walking around the stage holding both hands clasped over her head like a boxer circling the ring. It was outrageous. Patrick had no experience with handling a Hollywood-grown ego of that size and probably wasn't very good at it. Also, there was the frustration of having been part of something that had worked so well, been such a wonderful experience, that had now become a battlefield of nerves and tension. So it was not the great time we thought it would be.

Then one night, a couple of months into the run, Patrick came home from the theater bringing five other actors with him—some from *Iguana*, some from the O'Neill play down the street. I'd gotten used to late-night unexpected guests so I was prepared—plenty of food and drink on hand. Some of these after-theater suppers had been great fun: interesting people, lots of theater stories, and me running in and out of the kitchen. But that night was not fun. After everyone else left, one of the actors stayed on, and he and Patrick kept drinking. I had never seen my husband drink that way before.

He was a man on a mission—he was flat-out drinking to get drunk, to get as drunk as he possibly could. The two of them were sitting there telling each other tales, so slurred of speech I could barely understand a word they were saying, lurching to the bar every few minutes to refill their drinks.

The next thing I remember about that night was being in my bathroom in the dark—sitting on the edge of the bathtub tightly wrapped in my own two arms. Our apartment was on the nineteenth floor, and out the window was a great expanse of black night sky. I stared out at a million stars as I slowly rocked back and forth, my own voice whispering in the darkness, "Something terrible is happening."

"Something terrible is happening . . ."

I was absolutely right. That night was the beginning. After that Patrick got more and more drunk, more and more often. I didn't know what to do. I didn't understand anything about the disease of addiction. All I really did was feel frightened and miserable. Well, that and judge, criticize, and berate. It was not a good time, and it accelerated over the next few years. Finally, the inevitable: Patrick went out to LA to film something, I don't remember what, and was fired from the job. He'd arrived on the set one morning very late and very hungover. Fortunately there was another actor on the film who was from New York, a longtime acquaintance of Patrick's and a recovering alcoholic himself. He told Patrick to let him know if he wanted help. Wisely Patrick said yes—being fired had shocked him out of his denial about how bad things were—and that friend took him to his first AA meeting. The problem didn't get fixed then and there, but it did get Patrick more or less pointed in the right direction. After a few more disasters, Patrick did stop drinking and got some real Alcoholics Anonymous sobriety under his belt.

So Patrick got sober—but I did not. Like many before me and many to follow, I told myself that every problem we had was a result of Patrick's drinking, and if that just stopped, everything would be fine. Certainly nothing that wasn't working had anything to do with me! Of course not—I wasn't yet paying attention.

There was an incident that occurred one evening during that time when Patrick was sober that has stuck in my mind all these years because it seems such a perfect illustration of how unconscious I was in those days. At Friends In Deed we frequently talk about having compassion for the mistakes people make because, no matter how bad it may look, people are always doing the best they can at that moment. I do know that that was true of me back then—the way I handled that particular situation was the best I could do at the time. It just looks mighty poor from where I stand now.

We were dressing to go out. The party we were going to would be small and celebrity filled. I was looking in a drawer for the earrings I wanted to wear. Patrick walked into the room behind me, and I heard him ask, "Why do you think they've invited us? Why are we asked to these things?"

My heart sank. I knew exactly what he was asking.

Evenings like the one we were headed for were fun and completely comfortable for me. Sometimes they weren't for Patrick.

Was it difficult for Patrick to be with other people who were so much more successful than he was, in a worldly sense? Was it particularly hard because he had so slowed the upward trajectory of his own career with drugs and alcohol? I think the answer to both questions would be yes.

Of course you would never have known it to look at him. He had a black belt in cool, my Patrick did—and wit. He could wait it out and wait it out and then say the wittiest thing of the night on his way out the door.

So even though I knew he didn't feel just fine that night, he looked just fine—in fact, particularly fine: dark blue Sills suit, creamy English shirt, brilliant yellow silk tie.

Our marvelous housekeeper, Loretta, used to say to me, "Oh, look at that man! Doesn't he look like some king of the land?" She also used to say to me, "Honey, you're lucky I make your side of the bed!"

So the question: Why us? I answered by joking that I should think we'd been asked because we're both so very darling. I quoted Scott Fitzgerald's little poem:

The people all clapped
As we arose
For her sweet face
And my new clothes.

I had lightly skimmed right past what I knew in my heart—afraid that if we really talked about it some changes would have to be made that I didn't want to make. I wanted to keep going to those parties.

Patrick answered in kind: "Well, you're lookin' good, kid. Lookin' good!"

On a summer weekend in 1972 Patrick and I had the most heated argument we'd had in a long, long time. We were at our recently acquired country house in Cold Spring Harbor on the North Shore of Long Island. Patrick told me that he was going to do the est training, and I responded by going completely berserk.

There I was on one of those beautiful late summer days that has just a whisper of fall about it, storming up and down our big wide porch: "Are you out of your mind? One of those absurd California New Age fads?! Sit in a room with 150 creepy people? I'd rather kill myself! You're going to give up two beautiful weekends in the country to be with a bunch of New Age assholes?!"

Patrick's answer: "Yes, that's what I'm going to do."

Several people he knew in AA had done it, and there was something he was seeing that intrigued him.

Hard to imagine why he wouldn't rather be with me.

The argument raged on and on, me a whirling dervish, Patrick holding firm.

So on a Saturday in September, Patrick went off early in the morning to begin the est training. At the end of the weekend it was clear he'd had an extraordinary experience, but in his wisdom he did nothing to try to sell me on it. He didn't have to because just looking and listening, I could see that something in him had definitely shifted. It became clear that he knew something I did not know, and it was becoming very uncomfortable. Then one night at a dinner with friends, someone asked him about est and said that they could never do it because they couldn't bear being verbally confronted before a room full of people. Patrick told them that they didn't have to be. People only talked if they raised their hand—you never had to say a word if you didn't want to.

Oh. I hadn't known that.

A few days later I remarked that even if one didn't choose to raise one's hand, it still must be a very scary room to be in. Patrick said, "It's the safest place I've ever been."

Coming from Patrick, that was an amazing sentence. What had happened in those four days that had so changed Patrick? Much as I was attached to my idea of myself as a person who loathed such things, who wouldn't be caught dead doing anything that could possibly be referred to as New Age, my curiosity finally got the better of me and I had to see for myself what went on in that room. Feeling slightly embarrassed about it, I signed up for the next available training. I'm not sure that I even told anyone other than Patrick what I was doing.

At one point during the training it occurred to me that what was happening was rather like standing next to a car with the hood raised while a brilliant mechanic explained, with great clarity and precision, just how an engine works, what exactly makes a car run. In this case Werner Erhard was the mechanic, and what he was teaching us was how people "work," how life "works." First a concept would be presented, which by definition would be interesting but cerebral. Then, in the dialogue that followed while people questioned or disagreed with the concept, we saw the premise being proved right before our eyes. It became experiential.

In hindsight it seems to me that est was simply saying exactly what we have heard from every wise teacher and thinker through the ages. William James said, "The greatest discovery of my generation is that human beings can alter their lives by altering their attitudes of mind." In the Talmud it says, "We do not see things as they are. We see them as *we* are." Proust said, "The real voyage of discovery consists not in seeking new landscapes but in having new eyes." Sophocles said, "The greatest griefs are those we cause ourselves." Marcus Aurelius said, "Our life is what our thoughts make of it." Agnes Repplier said, "It is not easy to find happiness in ourselves, and it is not possible to find it elsewhere." Voltaire said, "Each player must accept the cards life deals him or her. But once they are in hand, he or she alone must decide how to play the cards in order to win the game." Hazrat Inayat Khan said, "Life is what it is, you cannot change it, but you can change yourself." Shakespeare said, "There is nothing either bad nor good but thinking makes it so." In short, the whole thing is an inside job.

Other people might say est was about something else, I don't know. For me, that was the heart of the matter, and it changed everything. I had been sure that if I could just get everything in my external material world just the way I wanted it—all the pieces on the board in exactly the right squares—I'd be happy. Werner showed me that neither happiness nor unhappiness is *ever* in the circumstance. What was remarkable about it was that he didn't just tell us that's how it works—he demonstrated it. Over and over again, as the trainer worked with one of the participants, it became clear that it wasn't the circumstance that was causing the misery—it was the way they viewed the circumstance—how they were holding it. We see it at Friends In Deed all the time, ten different people with cancer—ten different experiences. It's not what happens, it's what we do with what happens.

That principle was shown to us again and again in the course of those two weekends. There were other things to be learned, other nuances, but for me that was the big one. While there are things outside myself I am powerless to change, I can change my perception of them—and that's all I have to change. That powerful teaching is the very backbone of the work we do at Friends In Deed.

Beyond the actual est training, Patrick and I spent a fair amount of time around Werner, and it was always clear to me that I was in the presence of an extraordinary mind and that what I had learned from him was a gift that would last me all my life. Once when Patrick was in Ireland as a guest of John Huston, the other houseguest was Buckminster Fuller. During their time together, they spoke of Werner. Mr. Fuller had given several lectures in partnership with Werner, and he told Patrick that there was no one with whom he'd rather have a conversation—there was no better mind, no more enlightened view.

I didn't realize it at the time, but what Werner had really done was to take the essence of Eastern spirituality and put it into Western language—very tough, very accessible Western language.

Werner had gone to India, trekked about the Himalayas, and spent time with various spiritual masters, all of which resulted in his bringing to this country an Indian yogi named Baba Muktananda. Muktananda ended up having ashrams both in South Fallsburg, New York, and Santa Monica, California, as well as the one in Ganeshpuri, India. It was Werner who first introduced this country to Baba and who organized the first events where one could be with this yogi master.

Patrick and I went to such an event, and while I certainly felt that I was in the presence of a wonderful man, I did not feel impelled to drop my present life, follow Muktananda to the baked earth of India, and sit around the fire pounding out handmade *chapatis*. Patrick was more drawn to all of it than I. He was, in general, far more a "seeker." I'm sure his being an alcoholic was a big part of it. Being happy was far more difficult for Patrick than it was for me. I don't know if I would have done any of those things had he not led the way. A big factor for me, at first, was simply wanting to share with him the things that he was drawn to because I was so thrilled that he was drawn to anything other than booze and drugs. Then I became genuinely interested in what I was learning. However, I always had a problem with a lot of the exterior trappings and still do. In any event Patrick was interested enough that when the ashram in South Fallsburg was established, he went to several weekend retreats. I no longer became hysterical when he made such plans.

On one of the weekends I said I'd go with him, and we decided to take Max, who was about five at the time. When we arrived, we found that Patrick's celebrity had earned us some special treatment. The guru was a watcher of television, and he had seen Patrick on numerous shows, so we were told that we might have a semiprivate audience with Baba. At the appointed hour we were to meet with him under a magnificent big tree with two or three other people and his translator.

Actually, it was the walk to the tree that I will never forget. Patrick and I had gotten into a fierce argument earlier that morning. I have no idea what it was about, but there we were, walking down a beautiful flower-edged path, hurling furious whispered remarks at each other. Finally Max, who was a bit ahead of us, turned around and flipped his parents the finger. Now, the glorious absurdity of the situation hit us. The oh-so-spiritual O'Neal family, heading for the guru, ready to kill one another—all love and light.

Sitting under the tree, I felt I was the unenlightened dud of the group. I was perfectly content to be there, but I was not transported as Patrick seemed to be and, to my wonder, so was Max. Our little boy could not take his eyes off Muktananda's face, nor his hand off Baba's knee. Within five minutes he was asking Baba if he could visit him in India.

A couple of weeks later I was driving Max through the countryside on the North Shore of Long Island. Max, from babyhood, was a rocker. He would throw himself back and forth against whatever seat he was in, and he always did so in the car. This time as he rocked he added the Alka Seltzer jingle to his rocking: "Plop, plop, fizz, fizz . . . Oh, what a relief it is! Plop, plop, fizz, fizz . . . Oh, what a relief it is!"—mile after mile. Finally I asked him if he could please sing something else before I lost my mind.

His answer: "I can't. It's my mantra Baba gave me."

Exploring various spiritual disciplines became part of our everyday life. Patrick's bedside table was stacked with Krishnamurti and Elmore Leonard, mine with the Tibetan Book of the Dead and Turgenev. We were serious but not obsessed.

Then, around that time, I met a spiritual teacher of my own. Channel 13 was doing a series of interviews with various religious and spiritual leaders, and they asked Patrick to participate in an interview with a man called Ram Dass. We knew something about him in his former life. His name had been Richard Alpert, he was a psychology professor at Harvard, and along with Timothy Leary, he had been asked to leave Harvard as a result of the LSD experiments they were conducting, which involved some of the students. We had no idea what he had done since leaving Harvard, but obviously, somewhere along the way he had become Ram Dass.

When Patrick got home from doing the interview, he looked like he'd swallowed a lightbulb. I tried to get him to explain to me what had happened, what it was. But as with Muktananda, he couldn't. He just kept saying that he'd never been with anyone like that, but he couldn't describe what "like that" was. He just kept grinning. Not too long after that, Ram Dass gave a lecture in the Hunter College auditorium, so that was my chance to see for myself.

There's a saying, "When the student is ready, the teacher will appear."

When I saw Ram Dass that first time, I sat there thinking, *Oh, so that's what it can look like!* Ram Dass is sharp, fast, articulate, wildly funny, and very wise. He takes himself lightly. Also he's an American; I could identify, I didn't have to deal with the barrier of red dots and saffron robes. After the drug experiments, Ram Dass became intrigued with the idea that it might be possible to get to where he'd gotten on drugs—without the drugs. Maybe you could get to the "high" without artificial means and without having to come "down." His search took him to India, where he began a serious spiritual practice and found his guru, Neem Karoli Baba. His lifelong work had begun.

One of my favorite stories that Ram Dass tells is about the time he went to the ashram in India and meditated, simply observing his own breath, for eighteen hours a day, for two months. When it was over he thought that now he was really there, he was "free!" He felt he was floating above the ground, he'd let go of all earthly attachments. Then he boarded the train to come home, sat down, looked

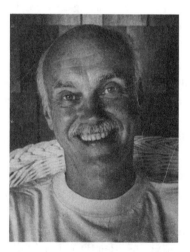

across the aisle, and was instantly and completely overwhelmed by lust. Now, this was someone I could relate to!

It was from Ram Dass that I learned about kindness, compassion, and acceptance. These were, of course, qualities I knew were desirable, but watching and listening to Ram Dass I saw that it was essential that I get to work on myself in these regards, especially the business of acceptance—of myself as well as others. Once, when he was visiting Friends In Deed, Ram Dass spoke of all the years he had spent searching and studying: He himself was a psychology professor at Harvard, had gone through extensive analysis, found and studied with his guru, had meditated and chanted for months at a time, studied the sacred writings of many spiritual disciplines, and with all that he still had every single neurosis he'd ever had. The great difference was his relationship to them. Formerly they were frightening ogres who ran his life, now they were like friendly well-known little Shmoos who, when they appeared, he'd welcome in for a cup of tea. His words relaxed and encouraged every single person in that packed room—acceptance.

It wasn't that Ram Dass was saying anything I hadn't heard, but I could hear it from him so clearly. He presents himself as a teacher, not as a guru. He has no ashram, no devotees. He does have devoted students.

After the initial lecture that Patrick took me to, I proceeded to put myself in any room that Ram Dass was in, whenever possible. There were talks, seminars, and weekend retreats. Then, several years ago, Ram Dass had a very serious stroke which left him in a wheelchair without the use of his right side. His mind and speech are intact, but traveling and lecturing became difficult and exhausting. Now he seems to have retired to a new home in Hawaii, so I don't know if I'll see him again. Fortunately he has written several books and made dozens of tapes on every possible subject. I have access. I carry what I've learned from him always. Ram Dass taught me about acceptance and patience. He also taught me that we are all here—a gathering of souls—doing the very best we can with the predicament that is life. Ram Dass taught me compassion. He is with us at every single group I facilitate at Friends In Deed. Actually, before his stroke Ram Dass came to Friends In Deed and spoke to us several times. In a sense I consider him our patron saint.

A few years ago I was at one of his retreats, along with a couple I had seen at many Ram Dass events. They are smart, compassionate people, both in the medical profession, and I like and admire them very much. They were telling us that they were soon off to India, to backpack the trail that had been walked by Ram Dass's guru, Neem Karoli Baba. For a moment I was awed by their commitment and I thought, *Oh, now that's a really great thing to do—I should do that!* But the truth is, it's exactly like my seeing the movie *Shine* and thinking that I absolutely must practice the piano every day, or sitting in an Italian restaurant, overhearing a customer speak fluent Italian to the waiter, and thinking, *I've really got to get back to studying Italian seriously!* These thoughts are fleeting—they last five minutes at best.

I feel a bit guilty sometimes. In the world of spiritual teachings I see myself as a kind of cat burglar. I scale the wall, sneak in through the French doors, quickly scan the room, grab the most valuable gems, stuff them into my knapsack—then I rush back out into the night.

There have been other teachers as well, but Werner Erhard and Ram Dass are the two who have had the most profound effect on me—the two that I am "channeling" most often whenever I lead a Big Group at Friends In Deed. To my listening they are saying exactly the same thing. The language of one is more pragmatic and harsh, the other softer and more compassionate. But they have been my teachers, my education. What I have learned from them and other spiritual teachers are my credentials. Well, that and my noisy life.

CHAPTER 14

When I walk around the streets of New York City, looking at and listening to what surrounds me, I often find myself whispering, "Oh, thank you Patrick . . . thank you!" I often regret that I didn't say those words often enough—good god, without his bringing me to New York, I might never have gotten to this city I so passionately love. But what I got from Patrick was not just a change of geography. I've been told more than once that the people who are most difficult for us may also be our most powerful teachers. This, of course, inspires both wanting to thank them and to kill them. In that regard Patrick was my greatest guru, and the work at Friends In Deed is very much based not only on what I learned from the people he led me to, like Ram Dass and Werner Erhard, but also everything in life with Patrick forced me to learn for my own survival.

We were married in 1957. By the late '60s Patrick's drinking had accelerated to a really terrifying level. We were at the point where social events were almost always a nightmare. In restaurants I would watch Patrick get up from the table and head for the men's room, artfully managing to pass our waiter on the way. By the time he got back there would be a new drink at his place, waiting for him. Or he would look across the room, catch the waiter's eye, then make a subtle little hand movement indicating "I'll have another!" Those evenings were an agony. I was absolutely unable to concentrate on anything other than counting Patrick's drinks. They clearly weren't that much fun for him either, and by and large he did his drinking away from me, came home in the wee hours when I could pretend that I was asleep and thereby not have to deal with a drunken Patrick. The next day I would have to deal with a hungover Patrick.

There was one particularly unforgettable incident in August '69 that was a perfect illustration of what our lives had become and how I handled things in those days. We had rented a beautiful little house on the cliffs above the sea in Montauk, Long Island, right next door to a house the Bernsteins were renting that summer. I envisioned a month of lovely summer days and nights—the beach, good friends, a jolly time with our two boys. There was indeed some of that, but there was also Patrick's drinking.

One night we went with Lenny and Felicia to the lobster restaurant up the coast, where Patrick got very drunk during dinner. I thought I just might die of embarrassment, and Lenny kept giving me looks across the table that were simply awash with pity. Then in the parking lot later, he whispered to me, "I really had no idea you were so brave, so gallant."

I was not sure whom I wanted to kill more—Patrick or Lenny.

The fight we had when we got home was as bad as any we'd ever had. I was, of course, giving him hell about his drinking, and things got heated to the point where a green glass lamp hanging in the living room soon had a hole in its side. I remember thinking, *Better the lamp than me.*

I felt absolutely terrified and helpless—I think if a stranger had walked in during that fight, they'd have thought I was just as crazy as he was—maybe crazier. Finally we did both go to bed, where Patrick fell asleep immediately and I lay staring at the ceiling with my heart pounding for a long, long time.

I awoke very early the next morning with a great start, an immediate sense of alarm. Patrick was no longer in bed, which didn't make any sense because by rights he should have a killer hangover and be down for the count till midafternoon. I got up and walked through the house and found that Fitz was still asleep in his crib, but Max wasn't there either. Obviously he and Patrick had gone somewhere together. I made myself a cup of coffee and walked around the house and yard, and as I walked I became more and more anxious. Patrick was absolutely furious with me last night—what state is he in this morning? Where is he? Where is my little boy?

In the early-morning silence, real panic and wild thoughts set in . . . the car was still in the driveway—they must have gone to the beach. Is Patrick in such a state that he might do something that would endanger Max?

Finally the waiting became unbearable, so I walked down the long steep path to the beach to see if they were there. When I got to the bottom I looked in both directions, and as far as the eye could see there was not a soul in sight. I was becoming more and more frightened when I remembered that whenever I'd walked down that steep path, I'd always noticed a rubber life raft lying in the tall grasses nearby. It occurred to me that I'd not seen it this time. I ran back to look and indeed—no life raft. Looking out to sea, I saw that the waves were quite high, and there was no sign of that little blue-and-yellow rubber boat. The sea was empty. Now any grip I'd had on my sanity completely fell away. I was sure that Patrick had taken Max out on that tiny boat and they were both lost and he'd done this because he was so angry with me. I should never have said all those terrible things!

Down the beach I suddenly noticed that there was a group of men pushing a small wooden dory into the water, and in the moment it seemed to me that this might be connected to Max and Patrick—that some alarm had been sounded, and now they were going out on a rescue mission. I dropped my unfinished coffee in the sand, ran as fast as I could up to the boat, and in a desperate attempt to appear something this side of a lunatic who should have her sleeves tied behind her, I asked them what they were doing. I don't remember what they said. It certainly wasn't anything to do with setting off to save the lives of my husband and my son.

I walked back toward the house, trying to think what to do next, gasping for breath after my frantic run, and then there before me, materializing out of the fog, came Patrick strolling along the beach, smiling, with our beautiful little boy bouncing on his shoulders.

I had not realized there was any fog. It was light and wispy and very deceptive. I had thought I was seeing at a great distance. I was not—I was seeing only a couple of hundred yards.

The feeling of relief melted my bones—I was weak with it. They were both alive. In that moment absolutely nothing else mattered. Once again, I slid right past how seriously dangerous things had become.

The drinking was now affecting Patrick's career. The word was out that O'Neal was a problem. The truth was that our whole life was coming undone, and I didn't have a clue what to do about it. It didn't occur to me to talk about it with anyone, I found it all so deeply embarrassing and frightening. I just marched ahead as fast as I could, chin up, stomach in knots.

Late one morning Patrick was stumbling his way back to bed after a trip to the bathroom, and I took a good look at his bone-thin, underwear-clad body. *My god,* I thought, *he's killing himself!* I suddenly saw how much weight he'd lost, how ravaged he looked. All my blaming dropped away, and what remained was just terror that I would lose him. The only thing that I could think of doing was getting him to a hospital—someplace safe. Patrick was obviously very worried himself because he didn't deny the seriousness of the problem, but he did say not to call our regular doctor, that there was a doctor he'd heard about whose specialty this was. He thought he remembered the name, and as soon as he'd had some more sleep he was going to call him. That is what he did. Somehow, from the recesses of his alcohol-fuzzy brain, he pulled out the name, Dr. Stanley Gitlow, called him, and made an appointment. Dr. Gitlow put Patrick into a detox hospital, got him cleaned up a bit, and convinced him he had to get to AA immediately.

Once Patrick was deeply involved with AA, I, of course, heard about Al-Anon, the program for those of us who did not have a drinking or drugging problem ourselves but whose lives were equally unmanageable around someone else's drinking or drugging. It was suggested that Al-Anon meetings might be a very good thing for me. But I, in my ignorance, in my arrogance, in my bullheadedness, was absolutely convinced that none of our problems had anything to do with me. Also, the idea of sitting around in church basements with a bunch of other women talking about our lives was definitely not something I was drawn to. The whole thing seemed far too pathetic for the likes of me. So I just kept on dancing and telling myself that if Patrick simply didn't drink, all would be rosy.

Things *were* rosier. It was a wonderful relief to be able to look forward to the next twenty-four hours without fearing some catastrophe. Then, too, there were all those various spiritual disciplines that Patrick and I were investigating together. So I told myself that I, too, was working, I just wasn't going to twelve-step meetings. No big deal.

Then, after being sober for almost ten years, Patrick got a bit sassy about his sobriety, rarely went to meetings anymore. I didn't really worry about it. I thought that those terrible drinking days were behind us forever. I was wrong. Patrick began drinking again, and this time was even worse. At rehabs they tell you that alcoholism is a progressive disease, that even when you're not drinking, the disease is progressing, that if you start again, you don't go back to square one. It will quickly be just as bad as it was when you stopped, and in no time it will be worse. That was certainly true for Patrick.

The next two years were a nightmare. Patrick would disappear for days at a time. Sometimes I knew he was sleeping—or more accurately, passed out—in his office; much of the time I didn't know where he was. He had always had a problem with prescription drugs as well as with alcohol, and this time I knew that he had added cocaine to the mix, so I was constantly in fear that he would kill himself with an accidental overdose or by walking in front of a speeding taxi or god knows what.

We were living in the Dakota at the time, and I honestly don't remember that much about those couple of years—I think I went through them in a sort of robotic state. I know that Patrick was simply not there a lot while I did my best not to think about where he might be. I remember that I barely touched the ground, I was running so fast.

There was one late night when Max and Fitz were asleep and I was lying wide awake, fully dressed, on my bed, simply staring into space. From where I lay, leaning against the pillows, I could see furniture, paintings, framed photographs, and dozens of different objects on the tops of tables and cabinets—all of them were completely familiar, the accoutrements of my life—and somehow I didn't recognize anything, it all looked dead. All life and energy had been sucked out. The colors were dulled, everything was flat, no shadows. I watched one of our cats cross the room—paw up, paw down—and somehow she was not the known cat, she had become a mechanical reproduction of a cat. For a second I wondered if I was going a bit mad. But the thought lasted only a moment—I have always known that for me going mad is not an option. But the fact that such an idea appeared for even a moment tells me how bad it was in those days.

Looking back on all that, I can't imagine how I kept going, why I stayed. But I did. Never in my life had I been on my own and I was scared to death of it, though the argument could be made that, in actuality, I was very much on my own in those days. But there I was, with our two young sons, in our lush Dakota apartment, hanging on by my teeth. Then, too, when Patrick was sober, he was so terrific. I so adored him, and I kept thinking that surely it would end—that the real Patrick O'Neal would return.

I kept busy, which is easy to do in New York City. There wasn't a lot of sitting about, wringing my hands, wishing my husband would walk in the door, alive and sober. I was always wishing for those things, but I wasn't wishing for them from a sitting position. I was running like mad. At the time we had a wonderful live-in housekeeper named Gladys; therefore I could come and go as I pleased—the boys would be safe. In those terrible dark days I couldn't bear being at home at night, not knowing where Patrick was or when I'd see him again. So I went out. I was an absent mom. I've often thought how much better it would have been for me and our sons if I hadn't been able to afford all that help. But I could. So I was out the door when the sun went down—anything not to be in that apartment feeling hollow and dead. The minute I wasn't moving, fear settled on me like a great heavy blanket that wouldn't let me breathe.

❖ ❖ ❖

Memory: One night when he was in his mid-twenties, Fitz and I were having dinner by ourselves at Pasquale's in Santa Fe. Fitz hadn't yet found his direction in life, he didn't know what it was that he really wanted to do, and we were discussing the possibilities. He began talking about what he felt his assets were, what innate abilities he thought he had to work with. He mentioned the fact that he felt he was very good at sizing people up—for example, he'd be good at things like knowing if people who wanted to adopt a child ought to be given one—he'd know if someone was going to be a good parent.

There it was—the question of what my son thought of me as a parent—there it was lying right on the table, in the middle of the rice and beans and chimichangas. I took a very deep breath and said, "What about me, would you have given me a child?" Fitz looked me right in the eye and replied, "I wouldn't have then. I would now."

❖ ❖ ❖

It was not as though Patrick didn't know that he was an alcoholic; he'd been in AA for almost ten years. Finally the day came when he'd had enough, when his entire landscape was dotted with smoking ruins, when he feared for his life and knew he had to surrender. He put himself into the Betty Ford Clinic in California. This was the first time that he'd been in a rehab, and while he didn't quite get the job done there (there was one more brief period of drinking and drugging, which culminated in a ten-day blackout, after which he had no idea where he had been or what he had done), his making the effort did make all the difference to me, and was in sense a new beginning.

Like most rehabs, there is a "Family Week" at Betty Ford, which the boys and I attended. I probably agreed to attend "Family Week" out of wanting to be supportive, showing what a good scout I was. I don't think I thought that there was much they could tell me that I didn't already know. I was dead wrong about that.

At the Betty Ford Clinic I learned that I too had a life-threatening disease—it was called "co-alcoholism." I learned that there was absolutely nothing I could have done to control or stop Patrick's drinking; it's not that I was stupid or incompetent. It simply cannot be done by anyone ever. I discovered that just about all the terrible, terrifying, hideously embarrassing things that had happened as a result of Patrick's drinking had also been experienced by everyone else in that room. The relief was staggering.

CHAPTER 15

Thinking about it, I don't remember either of my parents ever talking to me about moral values: integrity, patience, honesty, generosity, kindness, giving service, the importance of being a good compassionate human being.

I don't recall my father ever having a conversation with me about what was important and meaningful in this life.

Instead I remember fried-chicken-eating contests at Eaton's Restaurant, which I always won. I remember that when I had the worst case of poison ivy any kid ever had and spent days in my darkened bedroom draped in medicated gauze, it was Pawnee who sat with me by the hour making up funny stories to distract me from tearing off my skin from the itching. I clearly recall a night after dinner when I was about six years old, curled up on the sofa in the living room reading: Pawnee looked up at me from his chair across the room and said, "You're reading *Little Women*, you're eating a good apple, and you've got a loose tooth to play with—life may never get better than it is right this very minute."

The moment with my father that, for me, sums up our entire relationship took place in 1973 on a summer afternoon in California. I invited him out to the house we had at that time on Santa Monica beach to have lunch with me. Patrick was at the studio filming *The Way We Were*, the O'Neal boys would be outside all day running around on the beach—we could have a quiet lunch by ourselves.

When Pawnee arrived, I asked him to please drive me into Santa Monica so that I could pick up some things at the cleaners. We drove up the hill from the beach, parked right outside the store, and I went in while Pawnee waited in the car.

A young woman went to get my cleaning, returned with part of it, apologized for how long it was taking, and went off to try and find the rest. It was midday, the sun was beating down fiercely on the windshield of the car, and I felt bad that Pawnee had to wait so long in the heat. In order to distract him a bit, I went to the big plate-glass window and began making faces at him, then I started dancing around, lots of arms and hips—completely loony. People passing on the sidewalk looked startled, and I could see him smiling and laughing, clapping his hands.

Finally the woman appeared with the rest of our clothes, I paid her, and we drove back to the house.

I made avocado sandwiches, a Baxter family favorite, and took them outside, where we sat under the awning, eating, listening to and smelling the sea, sometimes talking, sometimes silent.

Late afternoon and time for Pawnee to go, we hugged and kissed in the doorway. He started to leave, stopped, and turned to me, his face full of emotion.

"You know how you were dancing around in the window this morning?"

"Yes."

"You know, grown-up people don't behave like that!"

"No, I suppose not."

"Well, don't you think you got that from me?"

I will never forget standing in that doorway looking at my father's face as he said that.

I suspect there has never been a parent more proud of their kid than he was of me at that moment.

My father would die before there was even a whisper of my current life and of the work I do with Friends In Deed. I'm sure that afternoon he didn't have a concern in the world about me—I'm sure he thought my life was perfect. I had a town house in New York City, a lovely old Spanish house on Santa Monica beach, my husband was at the studio filming a major movie with Redford and Streisand, I had two beautiful healthy sons having a wonderful time on the beach—my guess is he would have thought I'd surpassed even *Little Women* and a loose tooth.

What would he have thought about his daughter, who in his eyes lived such a glamorous life, throwing herself into the middle of the AIDS epidemic? I can't even imagine.

While there may not have been any important "life lessons," Pawnee did teach me to love art and to have great respect for all artists, to adore the witty (he himself was wonderfully funny), and above all, to revere eccentricity. In truth, those are lessons that have enriched my days.

My mother taught me some things that did not serve me well. The one great gift she gave me—a passion for books—was also the cause of one of the most embarrassing moments of my childhood. I had taken the plunge and invited my friend Jeanne to come home with me after school. This was always very risky because I never knew what I would find there. At the homes of other school friends, we would likely find a mother in a clean well-pressed dress standing in the kitchen of her orderly house, a mother who had already made tuna sandwiches and carrot sticks for our afternoon snack. At my house the breakfast dishes were often still piled in the kitchen sink, and there wasn't a carrot stick in sight. On this particular day Jeanne and I walked in the front door, and there was my mother, halfway down the stairs, wearing a rumpled robe, face unwashed, hair uncombed, with a book in her left hand, her index finger holding her place among the pages. The book was Evelyn Waugh's *Brideshead Revisited*. "Oh," she said, "this book is so wonderful I haven't been able to put it down all day!" I wanted to die. Of course, in retrospect it seems to me the most terrific thing in the world to have a mother who could not put down a book in order to do the dishes, but I certainly did not feel that at thirteen.

My mother taught me seduction—it was always implied that getting men to fall in love with you was the most important thing in the world. I suppose her fellow Hungarians, the Gabor sisters, would have agreed with her. She told me it was very important always to wear brown or gray eye shadow, never blue or green, and always to speak in a low voice. Those two things were, in fact, very useful teachings, and how much lovelier our world would be if mothers were still teaching their daughters to lower their voices. However, she also taught me competitiveness and envy, and those were not useful.

My mother said things that drove me absolutely crazy. If I made the mistake of telling her something I was feeling upset about, like the fact that all my girlfriends were going to the movies on Friday night and they hadn't invited me, I'd hear, "Well, darling, that's because you're the prettiest girl in the school, and they're just envious—that's all it is!"

When she said things like that, I really wanted to strangle her. I didn't know much, but I knew that wasn't helpful in teaching me to get along in the world. I vividly remember a day when the new *Life* magazine arrived with Elizabeth Taylor on the cover, and I said, "Oh, Mom, look at her! Isn't she beautiful?" My insane mother said, "Well, she's not as pretty as you are!"

I screamed at her: "*I hate to tell you, Mom, but Elizabeth Taylor is beautiful—she's absolutely gorgeous—and I hate to tell you, but she is more beautiful than I am. And I hate to tell you, but you are not going to win the mother-with-the-most-beautiful-daughter-in-the-entire-world award! Probably Elizabeth Taylor's mother is going to win that award!*"

When she wasn't paying me absurd compliments, my mother was nagging and criticizing me—it was one or the other, and it all resulted in my not ever really trusting her. Then, too, in high school I thought all the other girls were mean as snakes, so, all in all, I got off to a very bad start with the female of the species. Of course my only sibling is a marvelous brother. Of course my two children are sons. It is not lost on me that when I finally looked around and decided that it might be a good idea to be of some service in this battered world, I chose working with a community that was originally made up almost entirely of young men.

While I suspect my brother would say just the reverse, for me, my father was safe and my mother was not.

When Pamela came through the door of Friends In Deed, I did not immediately know that one of my most meaningful teachers had just walked in, but that was exactly what she and her mother and sisters proved to be for me.

Pamela was a very pretty young girl who looked like a Ralph Lauren ad and did, in fact, work for Ralph Lauren at the time. When she first arrived in that world of young men with AIDS, I assumed she was the sister or close friend of one of them. She wasn't—Pam herself had AIDS. My first reaction was enormous compassion for this lovely young woman living with that frightening diagnosis, but soon I was having a real problem with her—no surprise. The problem wasn't Pam. The problem was me.

Friends In Deed is meant to be, *must* be, a place of absolute safety—a place of no judgments. It's the very essence of our work, and I was having an extremely difficult time not being judgmental when it came to Pam. When she sat in on a Big Group where there were fifty or sixty people, she was too intimidated by the number of people to raise her hand or speak. But in a smaller group of eight or ten people, she did raise her hand, and always the words we heard were the same. It was all tragically unfair, life had cheated her out of what was her due (a long happy life complete with husband and children). All she had ever wanted was a "normal life," it's what she deserved, and now it was all ruined because she was going to get sick and die from this terrible disease. I had a particularly tough time with the "normal life" business, given that there is no such thing. As a group we certainly empathized with her—we also tried to remind her gently that no one arrives on planet Earth with any kind of guarantee as to length or quality of life, and it would certainly be easier for her if she could let go of the notion that life was ever "fair." "Fair" is most definitely not what life is about.

There wasn't anything Pam said that wasn't completely under-standable. You'd think I'd have nothing but compassion. I did have compassion, but there was something else, too, and at the time that something else was creating a real problem for me. I didn't think anyone else was aware of the edginess I felt toward her—I hoped they weren't.

I know at least a part of what I was struggling with was the con-trast. Here we were, surrounded by men who had AIDS, many of whom not only did not feel that what was happening was unfair but in the deepest part of them they believed this illness was something they had earned. On a daily basis I watched these guys, some of whom were so very ill themselves and had lost so many friends they loved. I watched as they took care of one another in the most com-mitted loving way. I saw these young men as heroes who lost another comrade every day. Then in came Pam, sounding a bit deserving, a bit entitled, a bit as though whatever was happening to anyone else, this definitely should not be happening to her. Maybe that's not even what she felt, but somehow that's what I seemed to hear. No, I was not doing very well with it, and I had to find a way to do better.

I know that a great part of my initial resistance to Pam came from places that were personal and historic. In one sense Pam was an American cliché—pretty, blond, a preppie-looking WASP; she would have fit right in at my old high school. The other two HIV-positive young women who came to Friends In Deed in those early days were of a very different cut of cloth—much funkier, not nearly so "normal." I didn't seem to have any real problem with either of them. But then they didn't trigger memories of San Mateo High School and the dread I had felt in my heart as I went up the wide brick walkway, up the steps to the big double doors, the feeling of going through those doors and knowing that in an instant I would find out what kind of a day I was going to have. Was I "in" with the gang, or had I said or done something in the last twenty-four hours that had me "out" with the gang? What would it be? "Out" could last for a stomach-knotting week or more. I just really did not understand how one was supposed to behave—in all those four years I never got the hang of it. I said the wrong thing, I went out with the wrong guy, I wore a red jacket with a yellow sweater in a world of powder blue twinsets. I was completely at sea, never knowing when I was headed for trouble, always off balance in a way that had not happened before and would never happen again. For me high school had been a four-year nightmare. In my view at the time all those girls who looked like Pam were more dangerous than a pack of wounded pumas. I could easily fantasize arriving at school in the morning, seeing Pam, walking over to her, and having her coolly turn away. Oh yes, I could absolutely see Pam doing that—just from the way she looked.

Then, mercifully, things began to shift. The more I explored the connection between my reaction to Pam and my teenage past, the

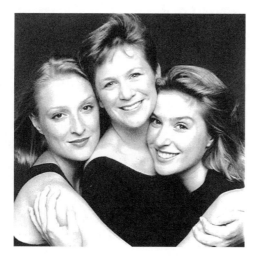

more absurd it became. Then, too, after awhile, we were not hearing so much about that normal life she deserved; we were now hearing about how scared she was, we were hearing about her bloodwork, which seemed to be very poor indeed—she said she had *no* T-cells. Was that possible? None at all? No T-cells meant she had an almost nonexistent immune system, and any infection could be devastating. We were hearing about all the ways in which she could see how terribly worried and frightened her family was and how painful that was for her. In fact soon her family became her main concern.

Finally what everyone dreaded happened: Pam was diagnosed with lymphoma. She'd been feeling terrible for some time, and her doctor finally hospitalized her for extensive tests, which revealed a very serious cancer. Now she was in and out of Saint Vincent's on a regular basis. The oncologist put her on a fierce chemotherapy regime, during which she stayed at her father's house because the chemo was making her very weak and dog sick—she couldn't be alone. Her parents were divorced, and neither her mother nor either of her sisters had the space for her to be as comfortable as she could be at her father's house.

Since she was too ill to come to any groups at Friends, we decided to take a group to her, and one afternoon eight of us sat in a circle in the living room of her father's brownstone. I'd talked to her on the phone many times, but I hadn't actually seen her for a while—when she answered the door the change was startling. She'd lost quite a bit of weight and all of her hair. She was very, very pale, and with the weight loss the bones in her face were more pronounced. Her head was wrapped in a pretty flowered scarf, and in truth I had never seen her look more frail or more beautiful.

As I watched Pam across the room, she seemed calmer, more centered than I had ever seen her. I didn't know if it was because she'd reached a new level of acceptance or because she was simply so weak that "calm" was all she had the strength for. Her presence had a profound effect on everyone—there was no small talk there that day.

The other clients, all men, talked about what was going on in their own lives with naked honesty. They told Pam how glad they were to see her, how they missed her at Friends, how deeply affected they were by the changes in her—in her they saw themselves.

During the time that Pam was too sick to come to Friends In Deed, her mother and sisters came to the Big Group. I kept my eye on them, glancing at their faces from time to time as they listened to client after client talk about their health, what was going on with their bodies and their medications—how frightened they were. I wondered how they felt listening to other young people talk about what it was like to go through exactly what their beloved daughter/sister was going through. Some of the scenarios were very, very grim—worse than anything Pam had to deal with so far in terms of physical suffering. What was it like for them sitting in that room?

I quickly grew to be in awe of Pam's mother, Marijane. We'd had many other parents at Friends, and often the mothers, most under-standably, appeared to be nearly hysterical, were barely able to hold themselves together, were not able to see how they would live through what they were facing—desperately wanting to hang on to their child at any cost. Please, please, would we reassure them that their son's doctor was the very best doctor in the world and that he would save their son? Not a promise we could make. Marijane was different. Certainly she was very worried, certainly she was sad beyond all measure, but she was also absolutely grounded and real with her daughter. She was holding on to the passionate hope that Pam would recover, but she was always realistic about whatever was happening in the present moment. I watched the calming effect she had on Pam, on all her daughters. In her physical abundance there were no sharp corners to Marijane; even her very appearance was comforting—one would find protection there—a warm and safe mother.

One afternoon, sitting in a chair in her hospital room, I watched Pam rearrange everything on her bedside table—it was part of the routine we'd developed. For several weeks she'd been in and out of those Saint Vincent's rooms, and when she was there I'd try to see her every day; most of the time her mother or one of her two beautiful sisters, Victoria and Donaly, was there as well.

This one particular time, I remember wanting to tell her to stop fussing and lie down. Just watching her tired me. But I knew she needed to do exactly what she was doing. It seemed to me that the frantic organizing, the endless fussing with the precise placement of every object in the room, was her way of attempting to control something—*anything!* She certainly couldn't control the progression of the disease; the chemo seemed to be having very little effect on the lymphoma. She continued to lose weight. She was a little weaker every day. Her bloodwork was not encouraging.

As she moved things around the room, she asked me to talk to her. She would say to me, "Okay, now tell me again all that stuff you always say about what happens when the spirit leaves the body, tell me again how we always stay connected to the people we love, how we never really leave each other." So we went through it all again. I reminded her that she and her mother and her sisters were all connected at the heart, and that's a connection that cannot be broken—it's there for all time. I reminded her that it wasn't her physical body that they loved, it was her—her essence, her beautiful spirit—and that even if the moment came when her body was too damaged to continue, that part of her they would carry with them always. Bodies die but spirits do not, and her spirit was the most profound and beautiful part of her. Then we'd make jokes and laugh about the improved body she was going to ask for next time around—definitely thinner thighs.

The state of Pam's health continued to deteriorate. She'd have a brief time at her father's house and then be back to the AIDS unit. That happened more than once.

Finally the day came when I visited her and it was difficult to hold a conversation. As we talked she seemed disoriented—I had no way of knowing whether the confusion was being caused by the heavy pain medication, or if the virus was now affecting her brain. Even the doctors couldn't be sure about that. Unhappily I had seen that scenario many times before.

Even as confused as she was, it was very clear that now Pam's attempts at any kind of denial were truly breaking down—she knew she was dying, that it couldn't possibly be too much longer, and she was very, very frightened. It was painful to watch her fear. Because she was not very lucid, any reassurances rolled right off her—she seemed unable to absorb whatever was being said to her—not by me, not by her mother, not by anyone. Terror filled the room.

I had come a very long way with Pamela. As are many of the clients, she was my great teacher. From my initial antipathy I now cared about her very much—I left the hospital at the end of those days feeling very low.

Then, at one o'clock one morning, Marijane called me from the hospital. Pam thought she would die that night and needed to see me right away—she must talk to me. I threw on some clothes and ran. When I walked into the room, Marijane hugged me and then left so that her presence wouldn't inhibit Pam from saying anything she might want to say to me. We had one of our usual dialogues, only now, though she was more lucid than she'd been the last few days, she still wasn't tracking all that well, so we had to go very, very slowly. She asked me to repeat each thing I said to her. Also there was another difference. That night, more than anything else, she wanted to hear that her family would be all right when she was gone; she was the oldest of the three, and she was used to looking after her sisters, her mother too. She'd been concerned about Marijane since the divorce—she didn't want her to be sad and lonely. Along with all the things we'd discussed a hundred times, I reminded her that her mother and both her sisters were incredibly courageous, strong women, just as she was, and that they were also coming to Friends In Deed—we would stay in constant touch with them, we would always be there for them, just as we had been for her. This idea seemed to comfort her some, and finally she became quieter and tired enough that she thought she could sleep. She loosened the bone-crushing grip she'd had on my hand, I kissed her good night, stopped outside in the hall, and spoke briefly with her beautifully brave mother, who I could see was anxious to get back into the room with her daughter. Then I headed for home. I didn't think Pam would be leaving that night, but I did think it would be very soon.

That week there were four Friends In Deed clients in the AIDS unit at Saint Vincent's. One afternoon I spent some time with each of the others, all of whom were certainly sick but not in crisis. Pam was. After checking in with the other three, I headed for her room and ran into her sister Victoria in the hallway. Victoria was completely distraught. She knew now that Pam was truly dying. It could only be a matter of hours, and she simply didn't know how she could bear it. A part of her wanted to run right out of this hospital and get as far away as she possibly could from the dreadful thing that was happening there. The other part of her couldn't possibly be anywhere else. She moved away from Pam's room, then back toward the room, away and back, so that she was quite literally spinning in circles, a lovely tall blond American dervish. I started talking to her. I did my best to find some words, any words that would mean something in the face of such despair. As we talked we walked up and down the hall together, and she finally quieted enough to face going back into her sister's room.

❖   ❖   ❖

Memory: I am walking down a hall in San Mateo Hospital. The hall is wide and cool—dull gleam off the linoleum and glossy painted walls. There is a peculiar chemical smell I've never smelled before, a kind of sinister cleanliness. It is very quiet. There are several nurses moving with importance in their white rubber-soled shoes. No one asks me where I'm going.

I am going to see my mother, who has just had a hysterectomy—

for exactly what reason I do not know. When she told me about the operation, she said it could be cancer—that maybe she would die. Her saying that made me angry. She frightened me. Proper mothers don't frighten their kids.

I find her room—number 127. The door is open. I look in but don't take another step. I am paralyzed by what I see. My mother is struggling to raise herself in the bed, her upper body is twisted slightly in my direction, but her head is down and she doesn't see me. She looks puffy and pale, and a terrible moan floats across the room from her to me. I can't move. I can't go to her. I can be of no help.

All I want to do is get out of there. Never tell a living soul that I was there that day. Spin around. Tear down the hall. Run. Get away from the unbearable thing that is happening.

❖   ❖   ❖

When we went into her room, Pam, lying on the bed, was a heartbreaking sight. She was deathly pale, and her white medication-puffy body could not be still. She moved restlessly and constantly in her nest of damp, tangled sheets. I was reminded of having heard and read about what an effort it sometimes takes for the spirit to leave the body, and it seemed to me that that struggle was exactly what I was now observing. I looked at Marijane across her daughter's bed, so deeply sad but also still and calm—though I had often seen her eyes fill with tears, there were no tears right then—some incredible unbreakable strength was holding her together. I couldn't conceive it.

The other sister, Donaly, arrived. On one hand I wondered where their father was, on the other this mother and her three daughters seemed to be such a powerful unit that it seemed right that they alone filled the room at that moment. Other people, relatives, friends, medical staff, came and went, but none of them made much impact. I wondered whether I should leave. They insisted I stay.

The four of us circled Pam's bed, moving from chair to chair so that we could take turns being right next to her where we could most easily talk softly to her, whisper in her ear. On each of my rotations I didn't stay long—I didn't want to use up very much of the diminishing time—that was for her mother and sisters. For the most part I stood leaning against the wall at the foot of her bed, watching and listening.

I'd never before in my life experienced anything like what I was seeing—those three women, reaching and bending toward their daughter, their sister, dying on the bed. All so fair and blond, their beautiful faces so full of both strength and sorrow. They whispered continually to their beloved Pamela, told her repeatedly how proud they were of her, how well she was doing, what courage and dignity she had, had always had. They thanked her for all she had taught them and for how, thanks to her, they had all come together with a closeness they had never felt before. They told her to leave whenever she was ready, that they would be all right, that they would take care of one another, and that she wasn't to worry about them. They told her, too, that she would always be with them in their hearts and that they knew one day they would all be together again. They told her everything that one could possibly wish to hear.

Two nights later, as people so often do, Pam slipped away when no one else was in the room.

All during those weeks I looked at Marijane Shaw and tried to find my own mother. I compared and all I could really find in common was blond hair and high cheekbones.

What I saw in Pam's hospital room had no historic resonance, no familiarity for me. Once my friend Robert and I were talking about our own deathbed scenes, and I said that I somehow didn't picture a lot of women around me. Robert said he agreed—his vision for me was more like a scene from *Boys Town*.

When I think about it, there is one visual image of my mother that I truly cherish. It's as clear and strong as anything else, and it's from a dream. It was a dream I had more than once, and each time it was so powerful it did not evaporate easily in the light of day. In the dream we were in a bedroom, neither hers nor mine, a bedroom I did not recognize. The room was cluttered. There were masses of clothes thrown over furniture. The lighting was dim, lamps draped with silk scarves; there was a wonderful smell permeating everything, probably my mother's perfume, L'Heure Bleu. It was an intensely personal room, glamorous and sexy. In the dream my mother was at her most beautiful, most charming—my mother at her blond Hungarian best. The dream seemed to be about her giving me, endowing me, or even blessing me, if you will, with a pair of butter-soft, brilliant red boots— Hungarian dancing boots. She was so alive in the dream, throwing her head back and laughing with delight—something I rarely saw her do in life. I knew that with those boots I could dance and leap and whirl! It felt as though, with those boots, she was giving herself to me, passing on to me her essence and all that she wished for me.

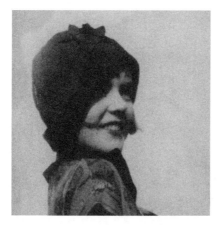

CHAPTER 16

It was the fall of '92, in the early days of Patrick's declining health, that we got a call from Bean telling us that Nureyev was in town and wanted us to come up to dinner at the Dakota. We no longer had an apartment there, but now Rudolf did. We knew he was ill, and we knew he had AIDS. On the long drive uptown from our apartment in TriBeCa, we talked about the night we had met Rudolf at our friend Christopher Allan's. Christopher was Rudolf's press agent, and he was giving this new Russian phenomenon a cocktail party welcoming him to New York. He was here dancing with London's Royal Ballet, and it was his very first appearance in our city. Standing in Christopher's living room waiting for Nureyev to appear, I thought I just might implode with excitement. We had seen him dance *Swan Lake* two nights before, and I was so enamored I was demented. I'd seen many other great dancers; I'd never seen one who brought that kind of danger to the stage.

Finally. Down the stairs—turned-out brown boots, Carnaby Street clad legs, that gloriously alive naughty sexual Tatar face, the scar on his upper lip that made kissing him seem a matter of life and death.

Nureyev shook my hand, smiled at me, told me he was happy to meet me, told me that, like him, I had "dog's eyes," which apparently meant eyes that slanted down at the corners. I was filled with joy at having anything like Nureyev—a connection. I babbled something inane about his *Swan Lake*. He turned to Patrick: "Is good to meet you—I like older men!"

In the elevator after the party, Patrick stood there looking at me with a very pleased grin. His out-of-her-mind wife consumed with passion and lust, and Nureyev hits on *him!*

As we headed for the Dakota, I though of other times in my life with Rudolf. I remembered standing, leaning in a corner of Rudolf's dressing room after a performance, watching him take off his makeup, when suddenly he stood up, walked over to me, and kissed me—really kissed me. If it had been the nineteenth century, I would have swooned.

I also remembered a night when Patrick was absolutely furious with me. He hadn't gone to the ballet with me that night, and he knew full well that I was going out to dinner with Rudolf and Bean afterward. So far so good. What turned out not to be good was the fact that it was a glorious night and, after dinner, the three of us had walked around the city—block after block—paying no attention to

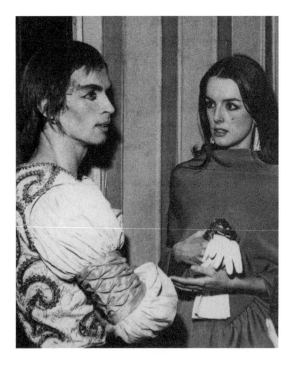

time. When I came in at 3:00 a.m., Patrick was not pleased—oh no, not at all! I guess it's wrongheaded of me, but somehow I honestly feel that there are some things that fall outside the contract—some things that you're not allowed to be jealous of because they are so obviously not of this world—like Rudolf Nureyev.

It's always been very strange to walk into the Dakota after having once lived there. Rudolf bought his Dakota apartment just shortly before we moved out of ours. Each time I went there to visit a friend, a great wave of sadness would crash over me as I went through the gates and thought about John Lennon.

When we arrived that night, we'd not seen Rudolf in a long time—he was based in Paris, and he hadn't been to New York at all for well over a year. He was here to conduct two performances of *Romeo and Juliet*. We had tickets, but I wasn't sure that I wanted to go. After seeing Rudolf dance Romeo so many times, seeing him conduct the ballet seemed too peculiar and sad. It might well have been different if he weren't so sick—an additional accomplishment rather than a reminder that he was too ill and weak to dance.

We had been hearing rumors about his health for a while—he had a very bad flu that just wouldn't go away, or later he had a serious pneumonia that was lingering. Then came the whispers that it was really AIDS. Of course, sadly, that made all the sense in the world, but then we were told that was all wrong and in fact, he was getting well, doing much better. I'd been holding tight to those reports—wanting to believe. Now, that night as we rode the elevator to his apartment to have dinner with him, we knew he was very ill—we knew that he did indeed have AIDS; it was not just a rumor. I'd been talking to Bean, and he'd explained everything that was going on—how sick Rudolf was, all the doctors and medications. It was unbearable. Of all the people I knew or had met who were infected with the virus, no one had been as much a part of my previous life as Rudolf—this was the closest to home.

When we walked into the huge, baronial living room, I was aware of several people moving about but all I really saw was Rudolf standing in the center of the room. He was wrapped in a long robe, Moroccan in style, and he had one of his beautiful small embroidered caps on his head—the kind he often wore as draft protection. His clothing was very elegant—ever the grand prince. But he was thin and pale, and as he walked toward us, his movements were heart-breakingly slow—he put one foot very carefully in front of the other. An old man shuffled toward us. We kissed, and I hugged a body that felt like a shadow of the one I'd hugged for all those years.

Bean was there and a few others—lovely Maude Gosling from London, whom I'd always thought of as Rudolf's surrogate mother, two women with heavy Russian accents I'd never met before. We all pitched in and helped cook the dinner. Sitting next to Rudolf, I tried hard not to watch him not eat the small bit of chicken on his plate—Rudolf, of the great thick steaks—washed down with glass after glass of wine. I kept thinking, *This simply can't be happening.* No one said a word about his condition, certainly no one mentioned the word "AIDS."

After dinner he and I sat by ourselves on one of the huge velvet sofas in the living room, and I thought that now he would say something to me about what was happening. He had to know I was safe. He had to know that I ran a crisis center for people with AIDS—if no one else, Bean had surely told him. But no—he did not name the disease, so neither did I. I took my cues from him. He did tell me that he felt dreadful, that there was no strength in his body—that right that minute he should be studying the musical score he would have to conduct the next night but felt so exhausted, he simply couldn't do it. He had no strength, no ambition. It was almost unbelievable to hear those words come out of his mouth, to hear him say he couldn't work—Rudolf who never couldn't work. Rudolf who could stay out well into the early morning hours, party the night away, then be in class at ten o'clock in the morning, not a minute late, going through his routine at the barre with such concentration and fierceness. But watching him walk across a room, watching each tender placement of one foot in front of the other, yes, I could believe it.

As he talked, I remembered once seeing him on a talk show. The host asked how he felt about his dancing—what would he do when he couldn't dance anymore? He said that dance was breath. If he could not dance . . . he could not breathe . . . he would die.

It was time to leave. Rudolf had gone into the bedroom and was lying across his grand canopied four-poster bed, having a massage. The door was ajar, so I went in very quietly, gave him a kiss on the cheek, whispered good-bye.

When we got outside the apartment, Patrick and I just stood there looking at each other, slowly shaking our heads at the complete outrageousness of what we had just seen. In the taxi on the way down to TriBeCa, we finally put words to what we were thinking—we would not see our friend again.

What I did not put words to were the thoughts I was having about Patrick's health and how pale and tired he seemed.

CHAPTER 17

As Patrick's symptoms grew worse and worse, we went to see a lot of different doctors. He was diagnosed with Epstein-Barr disease, and basically all any of them had to offer was the opinion that Epstein-Barr is all about diet, most specifically no wheat, no sugar. Patrick did everything he was told because he was desperate to find something that would alleviate the dreadful fatigue he lived with, the main symptom of the odd, rather intangible autoimmune disease— this disease that had us canceling almost every plan we made because he just didn't have the strength to go to the dinner or the movie or the theater, this disease that had me searching the health-food stores for spelt breads and sugarless desserts, this disease that had him lying on the bed for hours, shoes off but fully dressed. He'd get up in the morning and make a real attempt at having a normal day, get showered and dressed, and then after an hour or two he'd have given up. At another time having such a very different life would have been more difficult for me, but by then I was so engaged with Friends In Deed that I didn't really mind staying home almost every evening—which didn't alter the fact that I was very concerned.

The time came when living in TriBeCa did not work for Patrick anymore. Living that far downtown was fine for people like me who do well with the subway system, but Patrick's health had deteriorated to the point where he simply did not have the strength for subway stairs, and whenever he wanted to go to his office or to our restaurant, it was a very long cab ride uptown. Also, most of the time it was difficult to find taxis in that area. The whole thing just wasn't right for him, and I was okay either way. I like moving. Most people think moving is a horror, but I love it. I love waking up in a new space: It's the first day of school, it's a blank canvas, it's a brand-new life. I'll do it perfectly this time!

We found a beautiful garden apartment in a big landmarked brick house on West Fourteenth Street, which was built almost exactly when the Dakota was. Every inch of it had been lovingly preserved—fine details, wonderful old windows looking out on a perfect little formal garden, and in one of the fireplaces—though it's the last thing I would ever do in this life—one could roast a very large pig. Also there was a wonderful surprise element to this apartment. Fourteenth Street is a somewhat crummy, commercial, run-down street these days—its former glory dingy and dimmed. You tell someone you live on Fourteenth Street, and they're surprised whether they say anything or not—a very far cry from the Dakota. So our friends would come to that slightly grim neighborhood, then through a low wrought-iron gate and into what could easily be a marvelous town house off Belgrave Square in London. It was great fun to watch people's faces when they came through the front door. They were both surprised and relieved.

I think when they first heard our address, people often assumed the O'Neals had fallen on harder times. Well, we had fallen on harder times in the sense that my dear husband never really felt well and life was becoming increasingly limited and difficult. He tried many doctors, many remedies, none of which seemed to be doing anything. I certainly didn't see him getting any better. The only good part was that now almost all our evenings, after I got home from work, were spent having dinner, watching old movies, talking—the kind of hours when we were at our very best—always had been. If only it weren't that Patrick didn't have strength for anything more.

After we were settled into our new digs, things got progressively worse. Now not only did Patrick have no energy, he couldn't sleep. He'd never really been a good sleeper. He'd always hated the fact that I got in bed with a book, read awhile, closed first the book and then my eyes and I was gone. Now during the night he was physically agitated, couldn't lie still, got up and down, paced around the apartment, opened and closed the refrigerator door, drew another hot bath. All of this was something even I couldn't sleep through; I was beginning to join him in exhaustion. When I went off to Friends In Deed in the morning, I was worn out myself and very uneasy about leaving him alone. Patrick just didn't look like someone who should be left alone. I was becoming truly frightened.

I remember sitting at my desk—I'd just hung up from talking to Patrick—it was the sixth or seventh time he'd called that day. I hissed at him that he had to stop calling me all the time, I had to get some work done. Patrick had always been fine with being alone for hours on end; now he couldn't seem to get through an hour without needing to talk to me. It was irritating, but more than that it scared me. It felt as though he were unraveling in some awful, unnameable way. It was terrible of me to have been so short tempered with him on the phone. I wanted him not to call me so much. I wanted him not to need to call me so much. I wanted him not to frighten me.

In all our searching for answers and networking, a clinic had been recommended—one that focused on sleep disorders. The doctors there gave Patrick an antidepressant, saying that even for people not necessarily in a state of depression, these medications sometimes worked for insomnia. The first time he took such a pill he became even more agitated. He reported that fact to the doctor, who gave him a different version of the same thing. Finally he had tried four different medications, one after the other, and each of them made things worse as far as I could see. On the fifth day I decided not to go in to work. I didn't have a Big Group to lead that night, and I was so exhausted I knew I'd be hopeless at anything else. My brain was swimming in a murky sea.

Patrick had always been better at sleeping in daylight than in dark of night. Now even that didn't seem to be working for him. I tried for a nap on the sofa while he went back to the clinic.

That night Patrick took a fifth medication, and almost immediately everything went hideously and terrifyingly wrong. More agitated than ever, he was unable to hold still for even a moment. He frantically paced from room to room, me following behind trying to soothe and quiet him—impossible.

Then, as we neared morning, it became clear that something else was happening: He didn't seem to know where he was. He knew me but he didn't recognize our apartment. He asked me where the bathroom was, what room were we in now, was there a bedroom? Then he had the idea that we were in a *copy* of our apartment, like a movie-set version of the real thing. He'd look around and say, "Well, they've really done a good job, haven't they?" Glancing in the closet: "They've even got the right clothes hanging up!" He said these things as though he knew that there was evil intent behind what was going on—that "they" were darkly dangerous.

At one point he told me he wanted to look outside, so I took him out and we sat high on the steps while he looked up and down the street, not seeming to recognize anything. After a few minutes he seemed even more frightened, so we went back inside and paced up and down some more.

For several hours I'd been telling myself that as soon as the medication wore off, Patrick would come back, that his mind would right itself and I'd be able to reach him, to communicate and talk. The single ray of hope at this moment was that he did continue to recognize me and call me by my name. He asked me what the cats' names were. Oh god.

My own sleep deprivation was acute at this point, which I'm sure was making everything worse. Or was it? What could be worse than Patrick going mad? I don't know how else to describe the state he was in.

By midmorning I had finally admitted to myself that things were getting no better and I had to get some help—I couldn't handle this alone. I called Dr. R. and explained as best I could. He knew immediately that I could not deal with this by myself and that Patrick must be hospitalized as quickly as possible. He said that he would call Dr. G., a psychiatrist connected to his hospital, Lenox Hill, and that Dr. G. could get him committed to the psych ward, which seemed to be what was called for. It was impossible for me to believe that I was having conversations about putting my Patrick in a psych ward. What the hell was going on here? How did we ever come to this?

It seemed that, for various reasons, Patrick could not get into Lenox Hill until the next day, so some other accommodation had to be found for the next twenty-four hours. I thought about our staying at home and another twelve hours of my following Patrick around trying to keep him safe. I just didn't think I could do it. I had to get help.

After many, many phone calls, a place was found at a small Upper East Side hospital for just that one night. Though he was completely disoriented, when I told Patrick what we had to do, he seemed to trust me and trust that what we were doing was the right thing. He did not resist getting dressed and getting into a taxi for the ride uptown.

We arrived at the hospital and went through the admitting procedure, then were taken up to the ward where Patrick would stay the night. The ward itself was shabby, gray, and profoundly depressing. The other patients looked to be street people. It was impossible for me to reconcile to the fact that Patrick needed to be there—in that place.

But he did need to be there. He could not hold still for one minute. I was dazed with exhaustion. Whatever was happening to him was far more than I could handle. Patrick did not seem to have any real awareness of where he was—he just kept up his relentless pacing. I couldn't believe I was going to leave him in such a place alone and without me, but I was—I was going to walk out the door. Heartbreaking as it was to leave Patrick in that depressing place, I also felt real relief at the prospect of having a night by myself with the possibility of some sleep. The next morning I did feel slightly more prepared to handle whatever would happen.

When I arrived at the hospital, I found a much calmer Patrick.

They had obviously found a medication that had taken him down a few notches. He was quieter physically, and I was able to talk to him about going to Lenox Hill to see a doctor there—again he seemed to trust that I was making the right decisions. Was I? I definitely sensed that he knew he was in real trouble.

Lenox Hill Hospital was only a couple of blocks away, and I even felt he was in good enough shape that we could stop at a coffee shop for breakfast. As we sat in a booth eating and talking, I tried to explain what was happening in a way that would not alarm him. At one point he looked out the window, pointed across the street, and said, "Do you see those children playing across the street?" He said it with a funny little smile as though he knew full well there weren't any children playing across the street. I recalled that a few nights before at home he had pointed to a chair and asked me if I saw the woman sitting in it. That time, too, he'd said it as though he were being consciously funny—a wry little Patrick joke. It didn't seem to frighten him at all. It was rather as though he was somewhat pleased to be experiencing a kind of expanded consciousness that let him see more than I could. I skimmed right by the moment. I think I had been going through my days in recent times with my hands pressed tightly to my ears so that I wouldn't hear the alarm bells. I heard them now.

When we got to Lenox Hill Hospital, Dr. G. was waiting for us. We went into a little room where he interviewed Patrick. He asked those same questions I had heard other doctors ask FID clients: Do you know where you are? Do you know what day it is? What's your middle name?

"Patrick, do you know who the president of the United States is?"

"Well, now . . . That would be George Washington, wouldn't it?"

"Patrick, what's 56 plus 37?"

"Doctor, on the best day I've ever had, I would not be able to answer that question."

I was reassured by Patrick's irreverence and sass. Perhaps Patrick was, too.

After the interview the admitting procedure began. When I was alone with the doctor for a moment, he said to me, "Mrs. O'Neal, I don't think you realize how seriously ill your husband is." I guess I didn't appear frightened enough for his tastes. Dr. G needn't have worried. As the days passed I got plenty frightened.

The psych ward at Lenox Hill isn't shabby and dirty, but it certainly isn't a place you'd ever want to be. A lot of bare linoleum and Formica; nothing with which you could possibly do yourself in—nothing sharp, nothing breakable. The whole unit is locked and barred, only very brief visiting hours; patients wandering around with faces that look seriously troubled in some cases, blank and glassy in others. It is not a hopeful place. The only way I would be able to contact Patrick outside of visiting hours was via the pay phone in the hall.

Again, just as I had at that first hospital, I was going to walk out the door leaving Patrick behind. I was not allowed to stay with him; I could visit the next day for a few minutes. I wished I could see some alternative to the horror of it, but I couldn't. As the minutes went by he again seemed more and more disoriented, further and further from reality as though that walk and the breakfast we had together were just a sweet little window of light in the darkness. Taking him home looked to be a complete impossibility. The doctor said he'd had a paradoxical reaction to the antidepressants. They had tipped some balance; he'd had a psychotic break. It wasn't going away—at least, not yet.

I left the hospital and headed for Friends In Deed. It's fair to say that that day I walked in as a client.

As I rode the subway downtown I remembered several years before when Patrick made a film for PBS in which he played a mental patient in a state institution. It was filmed at a hospital in Reading, Pennsylvania. All the other actors were actual patients, and one day I walked over to watch the filming, which was taking place in a large fenced-in area, with maybe forty male patients all locked in behind heavy chain-link. I stood outside for a long time, trying to find Patrick in the restless moving crowd. Finally I realized that my eye had gone over him several times without recognizing him—so gray and ill and shrunken did he look. He had played that part brilliantly and now . . .

When I got to Friends In Deed I wished I could stay—just hide out there until the terrible nightmare was over. I was experiencing firsthand why this place we'd created felt so safe to our clients. Everyone was concerned and compassionate, but they didn't accelerate my panic—as opposed to Dr. G., my staff found my level of fear quite sufficient.

The next day that fear climbed another rung. The hospital had called me at home and told me that Patrick had become unmanageable and violent. They had to put him in four-point restraints. They warned that when I went up that afternoon, seeing him that way might be very upsetting. I didn't want to see him that way. I just wanted to stay in my office and concern myself with what was going on in our clients' lives. I'm good at dealing with other people's disasters. My own was another matter.

They were right. It was terrible to see Patrick lying on a table, tied down at ankle and wrist. I could see the violence in him. He had no idea where he was. He begged me to get him out, told me that "they" were going to come back and do terrible things to him. The look on his face said that the KGB was just down the hall. I must untie him so he could get away. *Please, please—hurry so that he could run.*

I was the one who ran. I did. I fled. I felt completely helpless. There was not a goddamn thing I could do. I talked to the head nurse, who told me that they had to find a medication that would calm him down, which they'd not been able to do so far. I didn't know what to say or do. I tore out of that dreadful place. Again I left Patrick behind. Life with my husband, particularly during the drinking years, had often been so difficult and painful, but I had never left him. I always knew in the deepest part of me that he behaved as he did because he was in trouble, and you don't walk out on someone you love when they're in trouble. Now he was in the greatest trouble he'd ever been in, and I was continually walking out the door. It felt all wrong.

When I got home I called a couple of friends and made a plan to meet for dinner—I couldn't just wander around my apartment all evening trying to get through the hours. Was this actually happening? Yes, it was.

I felt a strong need to reach out to our sons and tell them what was going on, or at least a not-too-frightening version of what was going on. I phoned both boys and told them as much truth as I could bear—I did not tell them their father had been tied down because at that moment he was a complete madman. Anyway, maybe the doctors would find the right medication and it would all be much better tomorrow. Dr. R. had assured me my husband was getting the best possible care.

When I got home from dinner I checked my answering machine, and there was a message from Dr. R. He said that Patrick had been moved out of the psych ward and into the regular hospital because it looked like he might have had a stroke. He'd call me in the morning with an update.

Call me in the morning? Now *he* was the one who had gone mad. There was no way in the world I could get through that night without going to Patrick. I imagined that all that violent straining against the restraints has caused something to burst.

I phoned Max and Fitz. I phoned Uncle Mike. I phoned our friend David, and we all ran.

Thank god we went to the hospital because actually, at that moment, things were a bit reassuring. We found Patrick sitting up in bed with a small oxygen mask on, much quieter, much more himself. We were actually able to talk with him. Also, now they didn't think he'd had a stroke—they thought he just had pneumonia. I was hugely relieved. People recover from pneumonia, don't they? I wondered why it was that he was so much quieter now—seemed to know where he was and said appropriate things to all of us. What had happened since that morning? There was no one to ask there in the middle of the night, so my questions would have to wait, but for the moment it didn't really matter. We were all relieved. The ball of fear in the middle of my stomach was slightly smaller. We could all go home and get some sleep—a small reprieve.

Lying in bed before I dropped off to sleep, I remembered that when I saw Patrick tied down in restraints, his voice had been very hoarse. I didn't think much about it—it seemed such an unimportant thing given what was going on. Now I wondered if it was that they had kept him tied down for too long without moving him around, and his lungs had begun to fill with liquid? Something else I could do nothing about.

It was a very small reprieve. The next morning I was awakened by another call from the hospital. This time they told me that Patrick had gone into pulmonary arrest and had been moved to intensive care and put on a respirator. They said that he was stable and was doing all right, but again warned me that seeing him in such a condition could be upsetting. I already knew that. I had been in dozens of ICUs and seen AIDS patients lying immobile with that terrible-looking though sometimes life-saving tube down their throats. Unfortunately I knew all about it.

I did not take the boys with me that day. I was as used to ICUs and respirators as you can be to such things, but I thought it could be very traumatic for them. Max had been terribly upset the night before just seeing his father with a small oxygen mask, which was nothing compared to what he would see now. I didn't think there was any imminent danger of Patrick dying, so I wanted to go by myself first and get the lay of the land—this frightening terrain I was pulling myself across, step by step.

For the next many days Patrick lay there, eyes closed, silent, unmoving, his body host to various tubes. They constantly monitored his blood for oxygen levels. All the testing seemed to indicate that things were moving in the right direction, but it was as though he had gone far, far away. I think he had. I don't think Patrick could stay around for a tube down his throat in the ICU. All of it was too frightening. So he just checked out. He went somewhere where it couldn't get him. Oddly enough, serious as the situation was, there was a kind of relief in seeing him lie still, looking like someone just peacefully asleep. I would stand there staring at him, feeling glad that he was getting some rest. Maybe all this deep sleep would be good for him, if you didn't focus on that tube.

I haunted the hospital. There was a small room for the ICU visitors. The reasonably comfortable chairs were filled with people who would go in and check on whomever it was they were there for, then come back to that little room and report on how things were going. There was a young woman lying in one of the cubicles who had several family members there, and we all got to know one another quite well. Everyone was rooting for everyone else—as though if the gods of recovery were present, it would affect us all. Hours and hours we spent together, and I don't think I would recognize any of the waiting-room people if we met on the street today. Friends of Patrick and mine would come to spend time there with me, which helped to ground me, but basically those hours and days had an out-of-body quality: The plastic. The hospital smell. The fluorescent lights. The fear. Like endlessly swimming around in some enormous watery tank. Actually the different cubicles that the patients were in were all glass walled, so that one could stand outside and look in as if observing fish in an aquarium.

After a few days they began reducing the oxygen flowing into Patrick's lungs and measuring how much he could breathe on his own. When the ratio was what it needed to be—I think it took two weeks—they removed the respirator, and then the focus was on his returning to consciousness. What if he didn't? What if the pulmonary arrest, when there was no oxygen getting to his brain, had done permanent damage? Sunny von Bülow—a new fear.

Patrick stayed in that far-off land he'd gone to for a couple more days. I talked to him endlessly, trying to coax him back—though I had been talking to him endlessly throughout.

Finally his eyes began to open and he was back with us—a cause for rejoicing. However, once again, he was profoundly disoriented. It wasn't really possible to be sure what was happening. The doctors didn't know. Were we back to the old disorientation or was this happening because, as the ICU nurses kept telling me, most people are very confused after being on a respirator for so many days? Also, look at the surroundings! All that metal and glass—how would anyone as sick as Patrick was know where he was?

Happily, Patrick did not seem terribly upset. Mostly, he seemed to think we were on a boat, and given how much Patrick loved being on boats, I thought it a very pleasant choice—why not prefer to be on a boat? It was certainly better than being where we were.

Medically he was improving. He began to talk quite a lot, none of it making a great deal of sense. Then one day his humor came back. He made a truly awful joke, and I allowed myself to be a bit hopeful. They had him sitting up in a chair with a sheet over his knees. Suddenly he put his head down and pulled the sheet up over his head.

"Patrick, what are you doing?"

"I'm feeling sheety."

When it was apparent that his life was no longer in danger, they moved Patrick out of the ICU and into the neurological unit of the hospital. The disorientation was continuing, and now the agitation was coming back. There were moments of lucidity, usually when I first entered the room or when the boys went to see him. But in general he was pretty much a mess. We had to hire round-the-clock attendants, strong young men, to be with him, just to keep him in the room, to prevent him from falling when he got up. He was very unsteady on his feet.

One afternoon at the hospital I left the room to get something, to make a call, perhaps, I don't remember—as I returned to his room there was Patrick standing in the doorway, holding on to the door-jamb for support, looking out into the hallway, calling my name, over and over: "Cynthia! Cynthia! Cynthia!"

As I passed her the nurse at the desk looked up and said, "Oh, yes—he does that all night long—he calls your name all night long."

"He does? My god, why didn't someone tell me?"

I decided to stay there with him in his room that night. Then I saw it for myself. He could not, could not, *could not* be still.

He was like some wild broken toy—some mad wind-up figure of a man gone berserk. I'd get him to lie on the bed, I'd lie right next to him and hold him, and before the count of ten, he was up again, prowling and fussing and talking nonstop—not making very much sense, saying my name again and again. I crawled home at sunup, exhausted and numb, powerless to quiet him.

I didn't try it again. I knew I had to have some sleep each night to get through what had to be gotten through the next day, and there could be no sleep in that room.

The days passed. Then one day Dr. R. took me out into the hall and told me that I really should start looking into places where Patrick could go, should he not get any better. It was clear that Dr. R. didn't think he was going to get any better. My mind bounced off of that sentence like water off a red-hot griddle. Certainly the Patrick O'Neal in that room could not come home, but what was being suggested was unthinkable. He simply had to get well. Of course he would get well.

Later that day I spoke to our friend David on the phone and told him what the doctor had said. "Okay," said David. "I know a great man, a psychiatrist named Sam Klagsbrun. I'm going to ask him to take a look at Patrick." The next day, he showed up with Dr. K., who was somehow reassuring the moment I met him—just something about him I knew I could trust. He went into the room with Patrick and came out ten minutes later saying that he wasn't at all sure that Patrick was lost, he thought the chances were good that he could bring him back. Dr. Klagsbrun was the head of a psychiatric hospital out in the country, and he felt that would be a good place to take him, that it would be very difficult for Patrick to get much better in the hospital atmosphere he was in. So that's what we did.

We took Patrick up to Four Winds, Dr. K.'s hospital in Katonah, New York. He stayed there for about a month. Each weekend when I went to see him, he seemed improved over the week before, and those weeks were a bit of a respite for me. I could have a somewhat normal life. But Patrick was never off my mind for a moment—I was always half awaiting one of those phone calls that would bring bad news. There had been so many of them. I had a running dialogue with God to please, please, please make him well.

At the end of the month I was able to bring him home.

Patrick came home in September. All through the fall he seemed to improve, bit by bit, day by day, to the point where we even decided to have a small version of our traditional Christmas Eve party. He went uptown to his office for a couple of hours most days, we went to movies, had dinner in restaurants—all of which gave life the appearance of some normalcy. But he was obviously fragile physically, and he phoned me at my office a dozen times a day.

That January, we decided to go to Key West for a week. It was there that the house of cards really began to collapse. Patrick had become fearful of many things. He had developed such severe claustrophobia that he almost couldn't get into an elevator. His first question about any place he had to go was "What floor is it on?" He dragged himself up and down many a flight of stairs to avoid the elevator. He was also afraid to fly, so we went down and back to Florida on the train. It was an exhausting trip—all that restlessness in a train compartment. I can remember a couple of nice dinners in Key West restaurants, sitting at the end of a pier watching the sun go down. But I also remember that I did all the driving because he didn't seem strong enough, and all the time we were in the car, he kept telling me to slow down and be careful, seemingly threatened by every other car on the road. I also remember that one day we went to a big drug-store, and for a minute Patrick lost me in the aisles. When I found him again, the look on his face was one of sheer terror. He said, "I thought I'd never see you again!"

The day before we were to leave, Patrick suddenly appeared next to me on the beach saying, "I think I have to get to a doctor. I think something's very wrong, I might be having a heart attack." So, we did. We got to a doctor, who examined him and couldn't find anything physically wrong but suggested we see someone as soon as we got back to New York.

The return train trip was even worse—more restless, more sleepless. As we were nearing New York City in the late morning, it suddenly got dark outside the windows, and Patrick became terrified. "What's happening?" When I explained that we were just going under the Hudson River and we'd be home very soon, he seemed almost to collapse. He had no idea we had to go down beneath the river! Why hadn't I told him? He would never have made the trip if he'd known we had to go under the earth like that! We'd left the city in the dark of the night, so this was a surprise—a terrible surprise.

Finally I had to admit to myself that Patrick was far more ill, both physically and mentally, than he had been when he first came back from Four Winds. I called Dr. Klagsbrun, and his suggestion was that we see a colleague of his who was connected to a hospital here in the city—New York University Hospital. I don't even remember that doctor's name—our time with him was so short. They put Patrick in the good old psych ward again, but among the preliminary physical tests they did upon admission was one that seemed to indicate he might have tuberculosis.

There is nothing that puts more fear into the hearts of hospital personnel than tuberculosis! They couldn't get Patrick into an isolation room fast enough, and those next couple of weeks were a complete nightmare. He was trying to get out of bed all the time, so we had to get people to stay with him again, but this time it was very difficult because now a lot of those strong young men didn't want to be in the room with someone who had TB, even though they would always be wearing protective masks.

They gave him the standard TB medication, brought food at mealtimes, which they left out in the hall without even looking in the room to see if there was someone there to get the tray and do the feeding. The internist assigned to him came every couple of days to check on Patrick's progress, and that was pretty much it. The isolation room was down at the end of a long, long hall, and the nurses never quite seemed to get that far on their rounds. I sat there hour after hour, wondering what would happen to Patrick if I weren't there, if we weren't able to have private nursing. My impression was that they would have just left Patrick there to die. That may be a bit melodramatic, but that's how it felt. That hospital seemed big and cold and uncaring. It was a terrible time.

After a few weeks it did seem that it would be possible to bring him home. The TB appeared to be improving, as did his lucidity. He wasn't well enough to be all alone in the apartment, but it was a time when Max was available to come and stay with his father when I went to work. In an attempt to get some weight on him, we fed Patrick all his favorite foods, mounds of mashed potatoes for one, gave him his medications and endless vitamins and supplements, and all the while searched his face and body for any signs of improvement. We went to the doctor he'd been assigned to at the hospital to check his progress. There wasn't much progress to check, but the doctor kept saying that it takes a long time for TB to develop and a long time for it heal—we just had to be patient.

When I remember those weeks, they seem to have a kind of film over them, one day and night blending into the next. I don't think I ever took a single deep, relieved breath during that time. Every now and then there appeared to be some small victory—or so we told ourselves—that indicated he really was getting well. But in truth anxiety was my shadow; it followed me everywhere.

One very clear moment pops out of the general grayness. We were in the kitchen, and I was standing at the sink. Patrick reached past me to get a coffee cup out of the cupboard, and as he did so, he said, "Maybe it would be easier to just die!" That was one of the moments I can barely think about. There was an opening to really talk to him about how frightened he was—obviously he was seeing his death as a possibility. I did not seize the moment as I wish I had. Instead I said something about how I thought that death probably was easier, that my guess was that death was just fine, but that I certainly couldn't bear thinking about life without him. I think there was some anger in the way that I said it—a kind of *don't you dare think about leaving me!* He turned and went back to the bedroom.

In the last week of May there was a definite decline. Then on Friday evening, on the eve of Memorial Day weekend, I came out of being with Patrick in our bedroom, thinking, *Things are going very wrong here. I've got to get help!*

I stood in the middle of the living room not knowing where to turn. I knew that if I called the offices of any of the doctors that I had been dealing with thus far, I would only reach their answering services; it being a holiday weekend, they'd already have left for the Hamptons, and I'd be told by some disembodied voice to take Patrick to the hospital emergency room. In that moment that just didn't seem good enough. I needed a doctor I could trust, a doctor who would be there *now*!

But whom did I trust? That was the question I asked myself as I turned in slow circles in the middle of the room. Then, suddenly I knew the answer—Paul Bellman! Yes, he was really an AIDS doctor, but certainly he knew about TB—many people with AIDS had TB. Also, I'd never seen a doctor as committed and dedicated as Bellman was. He took no weekend off, he was available twenty-four hours a day should a patient need him. He was a brilliant clinician. Also, he and I had a relationship. Many of the clients at Friends In Deed went to Paul. Even though Patrick wasn't HIV positive, I felt sure that he'd answer my cry for help.

When I called Paul and told him what was going on, he asked me if I wanted him to come over. Oh yes. Oh yes! He was there within ten minutes.

When he came out of the bedroom after just a few moments with Patrick, he said, "I think he's very sick and that we should get him to Saint Vincent's as quickly as possible." I went in and asked a very weak Patrick how he felt about going into the hospital. He whispered that he thought that maybe it would be best. We called an ambulance. Patrick was carried out of our apartment on a stretcher—another event that was nowhere in any life plan I had ever made.

When we got to the ER, they immediately hustled Patrick into a tiny isolation room where they put him up on a table and closed the door. It was excruciatingly hot in there. It was a muggy, steamy day anyway, and in that little room there was no air at all. Dr. Bellman was on the phone summoning his troops. He called the pulmonary specialist who he felt was the best there was, and very soon Dr. Larry DiFabrizio walked in the door and ordered immediate chest X-rays. When he got the results he came to me and told me that Patrick's lungs were very bad and so loaded with scar tissue that it was difficult to see anything. He also said that clearly Patrick was not responding to the medication he was on, and it was his guess that it was drug-resistant TB. Patrick was put on half a dozen different, very powerful antibiotics.

The isolation rooms at Saint Vincent's are all corner rooms, bright and airy. Patrick was put into one of them, around-the-clock private nursing was organized, and the wait began to see if the antibiotics were going to affect the particularly virulent TB with which his lungs were filled. One blessing was that Patrick no longer seemed to be agitated. For the most part he lay very still, not appearing to be in any pain, drifting in and out of lucidity. That whole month of June I checked in at Friends In Deed every day, facilitated my groups, and spent most of every other waking hour at the hospital. I wonder, how many times I did that four-block walk from our apartment to the hospital? Most of the time I was carrying food, Patrick was so thin, and the hospital food was certainly not going to get the job done. I had been told that putting on weight was a sign of recovery, that the TB was receding. I became obsessed with feeding him. If he put on weight it meant he would live!

❖ ❖ ❖

Memory: Something had happened that last April that I couldn't stop thinking about. I didn't want to think about it. I tried my best to shove it away, but, like those weighted rubber toys we used to play with at the beach, I'd punch it down and it would pop right back up.

When I did just allow myself to remember those moments in the kitchen with Patrick, I could feel my insides clutch, my whole body shudder. How could I have behaved like that, spoken with such anger, when he was so sick? So sick . . .

Patrick walking around in the kitchen. No, not walking—shuffling. Irritating sound of leather-soled slippers dragging over the tiles, like a very old man. Patrick shuffling like a very old man!

He'd just finished lunch, but not enough lunch. Said he couldn't eat anymore, couldn't eat anymore—as I watched his body melt away—the tuberculosis winning. Next he refused to take the handful of vitamins he was supposed to take at lunchtime. That did it. I started nagging and berating him. I couldn't remember exactly what I said. I only knew it was awful. Some really dreadful stuff about how hard I was working to get him well, and if he wasn't even going to cooperate by doing the simplest things that he was supposed to do . . .

Oh god.

After that he'd gone back to bed, and I was sitting in the living room feeling ill myself at the way I'd just spoken to him, the fishwife shrillness. Sitting on the sofa—paralyzed. Staring into space.

Finally I'd gone into the bedroom and told him how very, very sorry I was—how much I loved him, how deeply I apologized for speaking to him in that terrible, terrible way.

He'd said, "It's okay. You're just very scared."

❖ ❖ ❖

By the end of June the TB was improving. The regime Dr. Bellman's team had put together was working! Things were looking hopeful. Then one afternoon, as the neurologist was doing his daily check-in, Patrick suddenly began shaking all over. It didn't last long but it was definitely a seizure—amazing that it happened just when the neurologist was standing there. When the doctor went out of the room to order an MRI for him, I asked Patrick if he remembered what had happened. He opened his eyes and gave me a perfectly coherent answer.

"Of course I remember. It's just like what I did in *The Night of the Iguana*."

He was right. I could see him up on the stage of the Royale Theatre, tied up in the hammock, shaking all over with alcohol and madness. The two experiences had looked identical.

The MRI disclosed a lesion on his brain. It was right on the surface, easily operable. At first I questioned the wisdom of doing such an operation. I knew that the idea of brain surgery would be so terrifying to Patrick that he would opt against it. But he wasn't really cognizant except for a few seconds here and there. He could not be included in the decision, and I was assured that he would absolutely die without the operation. I gave the go-ahead. I felt secure with Dr. Bellman and all the doctors he had called in on the case, including the proposed brain surgeon. I was still telling myself we could save him.

Ram Dass often mentioned an Indian woman saint named Anandamaya Ma. He said that there was only one mantra she ever gave to anyone, no matter what the circumstance. The mantra was, "And this . . . And this . . . And this . . . And this."

Now I truly understood what she meant.

Patrick has had a psychotic break . . . And this.

Pneumonia . . . And this.

Pulmonary arrest . . . And this.

Dementia . . . And this.

Tuberculosis . . . And this.

Brain surgery . . . And this.

The surgery was successful, the lesion had been small. The surgeon felt he had been able to remove it completely, another rush of hope. After the surgery they put Patrick in intensive care for about thirty-six hours. Seeing him there was a ghastly sight: Patrick with his shaved head, long incision across the top of his skull, visibly in pain, moaning. I had an instant of wondering if I had done something terrible to him to put him through this. I stayed there as long as I could, talking to him, trying to comfort him. Then I was told it was time to leave, and I walked home with my heart breaking.

A few days later, on the Fourth of July, in the late afternoon, Dr. Bellman called me. The biopsy report had come back. The lesion on his brain was malignant. It was the kind of cancer that generally starts in the lung and travels to the brain. He felt sure this meant that Patrick had lung cancer, which they had not been able to detect from the X-rays because there was so much scar tissue from the TB, they couldn't see the cancer. He, Dr. Bellman, was not really surprised—he had felt that Patrick was not responding as he should have given that the TB medications were working. He was not in favor of trying to treat the cancer. He felt that putting Patrick through chemotherapy was unwise; the most it could do would be to buy a little more time, and the cost would be high. It might result in real suffering for Patrick, and right now he wasn't suffering—he looked completely peaceful lying in bed, never moving. He thought that we should simply do everything we could to make him comfortable. In terms of time he said it was impossible to know, but he guessed maybe a couple of weeks.

So there it was. Finally.

Cancer . . . And this.

Patrick is dying . . . And this.

I had walked the blocks from my apartment to that hospital, through the dense New York summer heat, times without number. I had walked those blocks in every possible kind of weather, but somehow when I pictured that short journey, I always saw it in the blaze of summer. Sometimes it felt as though I just stood there, my feet planted in the heat-softened pavement as Saint Vincent's moved slowly toward me—as though I had no choice in the matter. I had visited people in every other hospital in New York City as well, but it is Saint Vincent's that was a part of the fabric of my days and nights. Most of the people with AIDS that I had worked with had been there. Friends In Deed was twenty blocks from Saint Vincent's, that Fourteenth Street apartment was three blocks from Saint Vincent's—handy.

In the blistering summer of '94, I walked to Saint Vincent's day after day to be with my husband as he lay dying: to feed him, to talk softly, to watch our sons in their tenderness to him, to hold him— but not to hold on to him. That I could not do.

That summer has the quality of a dream—it does now and it did then. How could it be that Patrick was dying? We were going to grow old together. The joke was that we'd be in our nineties, walking along the edge of the sea—he with his splendid head of silver hair, wearing a slightly yellowed, slightly rumpled white linen suit—me with too much kohl around my eyes and wearing floating bits of this and that. The picture was so solid, so three-dimensional. How could it be that it would never come to pass?

Patrick had some very impressive longevity among his relatives— his grandfather, Doc, and his aunt Janie lived well into their nineties. Of course they didn't battle addiction to drugs and alcohol. They didn't have fifty years of cigarette smoke in their lungs. Patrick did.

Patrick lived another nine weeks. I walked through those weeks in a numbed daze, one foot in front of the other, not really knowing where I was. The thing that couldn't happen was happening.

Hospital. Home. Hospital. Friends In Deed. Hospital. Home. Hospital. Hospital.

For the first few weeks he was given steroids—I don't remember why—which made him ravenously hungry. He would grab my wrist as I fed him and move the spoon in and out of his mouth faster and faster. He was also ravenous for kisses. He would grab my face between his hands and kiss me and kiss me. Sometimes I would have on the orange mask that one was always supposed to wear in the room, and then he would kiss me through the mask. I did not always wear the mask. When his eyes were open I took it off. I could not bear the idea that after thirty-eight years together, his last looks at me would have me resembling an orange-billed duck. It was intolerable. The whole medical staff went crazy at the idea that I would do anything so dangerous, but I somehow felt that I was safe. I was not going to get TB. I had already been exposed to it for months before we knew he had it. In that instance, I was right. I did not get it.

Fitz, who was living in California at the time, and who has real fear of flying, got on a plane and came home. Max lived in Brooklyn, a short subway ride away. Both boys spent hours every day with their father. Fitz sat next to the bed, silently, just being with his dad. Max talked to Patrick constantly, told him that he loved him and that he was the best father in the world. Sometimes he'd get up on the bed next to him. Each in his own way.

Mike and Chris came every day in the late afternoon. Patrick's friend David sat with him for hours playing mantra tapes on the boom box. Another very good friend, Tim, came often. Other friends came to say good-bye.

I knew that all of it was right and proper, but the truth was that, as always, I liked it best when I was all alone with Patrick. I certainly liked our sons being there, but I really wanted Patrick all to myself for the little time left.

Patrick lay there day after day, rarely moving. Because he was thin, though certainly not emaciated, and because somehow lying on his back for weeks seemed to erase most of the lines in his face, he had never looked more handsome. When he spoke for the most part it seemed to make no sense, but I always knew what he was referring to. Again, much of the time, he thought we were on a boat. Often he was making a movie: "Do they need me on the set yet? . . . I guess I'd better get to wardrobe now!" One afternoon I knew he was playing poker with John Huston. Wrenching to see, he frequently mimed holding a cigarette up to his mouth and inhaling deeply. I had always been afraid that smoking would end in his having cancer. It frightened him, too, but that was the most difficult addiction of all for Patrick.

Every now and then there were a few moments of absolutely perfect lucidity. One evening I was feeding him his dinner, and he was altogether a bit more present, a bit more energized, than I'd seen him in awhile when the phone rang. It was Max checking in at the end of the day. After I'd reported on the three hours or so since he'd seen his father, Max said, "Tell him I love him." "You can tell him yourself," I said, and put the phone to Patrick's ear. There was a moment of silence, and then I heard Patrick say, so, so clearly, "I love you too, son. Have a good evening; your mom and I are right here." For one beat of the heart it was as though the two of us were sitting in our living room, and he was telling our boy that we were there if he needed us. And the world was safe.

Soon after that, he seemed to slip into a coma-like state—lying absolutely still on the bed, eyes closed, no sign whatsoever of pain—as though beautifully, restfully asleep. In one way it was a great relief to see him so—no suffering, no agitation. Peaceful.

I remember perfectly every word he spoke after that. There were very few of them.

Out of the silence: "Let's get on a boat together. Just you and me."

"Oh, yes. Where shall we go?"

"To a safe harbor."

Once and only once, he opened his eyes. He looked at me quite fiercely and said, "You know, I've done some very bad things!"

"I know. It's all right."

He closed his eyes.

Three days before he died I was by his bed, holding his hand, talking to him, as I did hour after hour. Out of the silence I heard myself say, "Oh, Patrick, I wonder. Did you really love me?"

The question just flew out of me. I hadn't even been aware of the thought. Looking back, I don't really know why I asked that question—but I did.

Then, strong and clear: "Why, I love you more than anything in the world."

Finally, the day he died, when I arrived at the hospital, the wonderful male nurse we'd had on many of the day shifts said to me that he didn't think it would be much longer. I didn't see any great change, but I trusted that he knew. Indeed he was right. Patrick died that evening. But sometime in the late afternoon, he whispered his final three words: "Patrick and Cynthia."

The night after he died, a group of us met at the Greens' apartment to decide on Patrick's memorial. We kept circling around the issue. Since we had no religious affiliation, there was no church or minister to run to. We talked of boats and the sea. We talked in circles.

Finally Fitz said, "I just want to be in a room and listen to people talk about my father." Yes, of course. Exactly right.

Ten days later we gathered at one of our restaurants, The Landmark Tavern, and people spoke of Patrick. For many it was revelatory. Both of Patrick's worlds were represented. The show-business friends heard about Patrick's life in AA—amazing testimonies from people who described how important Patrick had been to their getting sober—several people said, "He saved my life." The AA people heard about Patrick's show-business life. Both groups realized how little they knew of the other. I already knew most of the stories told by theater friends, but the AA testimonies were amazing to hear. Patrick had never said a word to me about how much he had helped other people—no boasting or taking credit whatsoever. I wish now that we had taped that afternoon, I remember so little of what was said—I was so dazed, no ground beneath my feet.

Throughout his illness there had been little moments when a thought that floated through my brain would shock me: thinking that now there would be enough room for me in the closet; that now I would have *only* healthy food in the fridge; that now I could do whatever I wanted, go wherever I wanted, without needing to seek agreement. Lots of little thoughts like that would dart through my mind, cause a quick gasp on my part, and then I would be flooded with the grief of losing him.

One late night before the final downward spiral began, I was lying in bed, just on the edge of sleep, when I heard a dog wailing—a real hound dog—*Aroooooo!* It sounded far in the distance, and it went on and on. I lay there wondering where on earth it was coming from; I'd never heard any sound from a dog outside that apartment before. Then I realized that it was Patrick. Patrick was lying there with a pillow over his head, baying at the moon. After a few seconds I answered him. So for a while the two of us lay there in the dark of night, *Aroooooo*-ing at each other.

CHAPTER 18

Grief is individual and personal. We have worked with hundreds of people at Friends In Deed who were dealing with the loss of someone they loved, and each person's experience is unique to them. There does seem to be one universal—almost no one thinks they're doing it right. Some people think they cry too much, others don't cry enough. Some are awash in guilt, some in anger, some in a combination of both. There are those who go silent and can barely speak and others who cannot stop talking. One of the things we hear most frequently is that they have friends who are telling them that they should be pulling themselves together and moving on with their lives by now. We live in a culture that is so uneasy with death that we want people to recover as quickly as possible so we don't have to be reminded that people die. We've heard people say things as crazy as *I know I should be getting over the death of my partner—it's been almost two months.*

When Patrick died, I was fortunate enough not to have any such ideas, and I was certainly encouraged by everyone around me to take all the time I needed. I was unbalanced and dazed in the beginning and stumbled through the hours—I remember that I had a couple of close calls wandering into moving traffic to the screaming of horns and the ugly screech of brakes. I was self-protective and ruthless regarding friends—I did not see or talk to anyone who exhibited even a whisper of feeling sorry for me. That I could not bear.

I could not sleep.

One night after leading a Big Group and then grabbing a quick dinner with a friend, I walked into our apartment—our empty apartment—and the pain of the emptiness, of the no-Patrick-ness, smacked me like a two-by-four. I immediately headed for the telephone to call someone, to distract myself, to get through the moment, and then I caught myself. I thought, *Wait a damn minute here—what do we say to people all the time at Friends In Deed?* We tell them that the only way to get on the other side of painful feelings is to go through them. "Feel your feelings!" we say. *Put your money where your mouth is, O'Neal.* So, much as I fought and resisted the idea, rather than pick up the phone I sat down on the sofa and just let it hit me. I don't remember exactly what happened. I know that I didn't cry. I wailed. I keened. I ended up lying on the floor curled in a ball. I had no notion of the passage of time—two minutes or two hours. Then the next thing, without really remembering how I got there, I found myself standing in the bathroom brushing my teeth.

The pain was never quite as excruciating again after that night. It was bad enough, but not as bad as it was that night.

There were some things I did that surprised me. There I was, a person who absolutely believes that what we truly are is a soul, a spirit, that we are not defined by our physical bodies. Yet, after all these years of operating from that belief, I still have Patrick's ashes and don't feel ready to let go of them to this day. I also still have a great tweed jacket and two beautiful Turnbull and Asser shirts hanging in my closet next to my clothes. I'm surprised by it, but there it is.

I was blessed. I had my sons, great friends, and Friends In Deed to help me through. I was constantly aware of how lucky I was to be able to go to a place every day where the entire philosophy addressed exactly what I most needed to hear. The staff was great. The clients were great. I was surrounded by the best possible kind of support.

The other great healing element in my life was the city itself—my beloved New York City. The life and energy all around made me feel safe. Often, on those nights when I couldn't sleep, I would get up in the early hours after midnight, throw on my blue jeans, and go out the door onto Fourteenth Street. Fourteenth Street is never empty—

there is always life there. I would just go out the front door, walk a few blocks, look into the faces of the people I passed. In the late hours of the night, the early hours of the morning, it was clear that there were others who weren't having such a great time either. A sense of—*Well, here we all are.* Connection. It would occur to me that if I lived in a less alive place, if I lived in some suburb somewhere, my grief would be unbearable.

❖ ❖ ❖

Memory: The ear-shattering sound of a leaf-blower brought me to the window of a very lovely suburban house in Brentwood, California. I was there on a short visit, to see my brother, a couple of old friends. It was the first time I'd left the city since Patrick died.

I looked out on nothingness. Costly homes with overmanicured lawns, empty driveways, all the cars neatly tucked away in their tightly closed garages. There was no human being in sight other than the young Hispanic boy wielding the leaf-blower. The streets were empty. At that moment there was not even a car in sight, certainly no people—no one walks in Brentwood. In short, no sign of life. I stood there wondering what on earth I would have done if I'd lived there when Patrick died. It seemed to me I might well have gone mad. What saved me was New York City when I couldn't bear my no-one's-here-but-me apartment. I am private. I like to be alone. I like silence. But I desperately need life outside my windows. I read in novels of those women who fascinate me—pioneering women who lived on the moors or on the plains—with no other soul in sight. Could I do it? I picture myself sitting in the parlor on a black horsehair-covered chair, my knees pulled tight against my chest, my hands holding my head in place trying to keep it attached to my body.

❖ ❖ ❖

214 | *Talk Softly*

A little more than a year after Patrick died, I received a gift—the name of the gift was *Rent*. On January 17, 1996, a young man named Jonathan Larson called me—wanted me to go over to the New York Theatre Workshop, where they were rehearsing a show he'd written. He wanted me to do a support group with his cast. I didn't want to go.

I didn't really know Jonathan all that well. He'd come to several Big Groups at Friends with his best friend, Matt, who'd been a client for a long time. Whenever Jonathan was in the room, I noticed that he listened to everything being said with what seemed to be great interest and concentration. When he called that morning, I felt bad because he had written me a letter the week before and sent me a CD with a couple of the songs from his show. I hadn't answered his letter, and I hadn't listened to the CD—partly because I'd been very busy but also, I guess, because I'd been assuming his show probably wasn't anything I'd be all that interested in. He'd said the name of the show was *Rent* and it was a "rock musical." Now he was calling with the same request: Would I please come over that afternoon and talk to the cast—the show deals with everything we talk about at Friends In Deed. He thought it would be of great value to his actors, and it would mean the world to him. I didn't want to go.

We were in the middle of a fierce winter storm. It wasn't beautiful, soft snow, it was ice and sleet and freezing wind. In short it was murder outside, and it was warm and cozy in my office, where I desperately wanted to stay. New York Theatre Workshop is in the East Village, an easy walk normally but certainly not in such weather, and given the storm it would be impossible to find a cab in either direction. I finessed making a decision by telling Jonathan that I didn't really give talks, I respond to questions, and he said he'd make a list of questions for me that he would ask, and then the cast could ask any questions they had. I said to call me back in an hour and I'd see what I could do. I still didn't want to go.

Sitting there, trying to figure out how to get out of it as gracefully as possible, a pesky voice in the back of my mind started up—actually, it occurred to me that what the voice was saying was exactly what Patrick would have said. *What are you thinking? Young actors doing a show about life and death and love and fear and AIDS? There's only one possible answer. The answer is yes.*

Later that afternoon, standing up to my knees in icy water trying to hail a taxi, I wasn't even bothered because I felt so moved and excited by what I had just experienced in that rehearsal room. We'd had a wonderful dialogue—Jonathan; the director, Michael Greif; the fifteen kids in the cast; and myself. Michael said that there was enormous anger around the AIDS epidemic and that anger needed to be in the show. Jonathan said that of course there was anger, but there was also something else, something he'd heard at Friends In Deed, and he wanted that something else to be there as well, so that's exactly what this meeting was about.

In response to specific questions, we talked about the insane relationship our culture has to illness and death—how death is regarded as something having gone very wrong, as some kind of failure rather than as the natural part of life that it truly is. We talked about how the whole focus in our society seems to be on length of life rather than quality of life and how crazy that is. Which is better—to live ninety-four years with most of those years spent in some sort of misery, or twenty-three years filled with aliveness and joy and love? I told them that the great focus of our work at Friends In Deed is on developing the fine art of living in the moment. The past is over; the future is fantasy. We support people in doing whatever they can to give each day as much quality as possible, no matter what the circumstance. We talked about the fact that no one arrives on this planet with any kind of guarantee as to their health or length of life. While of course it is particularly heartbreaking that AIDS is claiming so many very young lives, the truth is that very young people have always died—always will. We have to be careful that we do not let our focus on illness and death overshadow the beauty of life and our relationships—the things we should be celebrating. Some people seem destined to have very short lives—whether that life is ended by a drunk kid crashing into a tree, a bullet from an enemy gun, or by AIDS, the grief and loss felt by the people who love them is the same.

Also we talked about the fact that tragedy can transform people in amazing and wondrous ways, and how what I have observed in the gay community—the way people are taking care of one another, the fact that I have seen people who are so very ill themselves take care of a friend or lover who is even more ill than they—is as inspiring and beautiful as anything I have ever seen. There is a lot of heartbreak—there is also a lot of love. As I later discovered, all of this was pertinent to what Jonathan was saying with *Rent*.

We spoke of other things as well, but it was the part about life and death and love that was the heart of the matter, and as we talked I could see a real shift on some of the faces. They were beginning to look at the AIDS epidemic with different eyes. Maybe something powerful and transformational would be learned from this terrible epidemic.

I needed to get back to work, so I didn't watch any of the rehearsal, but I did know that something amazing was happening in that room. I saw it in Jonathan and those fifteen kids, but most of all—I could just feel it.

When I walked into Friends three days later, I stopped by the front desk to pick up my messages. There it was—a message from Anthony Rapp, who played Mark, one of the leads in *Rent*—he called to tell me that Jonathan Larson had died the night before.

It seemed absolutely impossible. Surely a great mistake had been made. Perhaps someone called about the death of one of our clients and the messages got confused. I immediately pictured Jonathan literally bounding across the rehearsal room to welcome me just a couple of days before. Never in my life had I seen anyone more alive.

I phoned the theater. It was not a mistake—last night, aortic aneurysm, found on the kitchen floor at 3:00 a.m. by his roommate.

Later that afternoon I got a call from Matt. His grief was so intense it was difficult to understand what he was saying. The most devastating part, of course, was the loss of his beloved friend. He and Jonathan had grown up together, they had been best friends since childhood. But also, because they had been so close, Matt knew what *Rent* had meant to Jonathan—how this show had been what his whole life had been about. Jonathan's dream had been to write a musical that would have a real impact on the Broadway theater, bring it into the present, and he had felt this production at the New York Theatre Workshop had a real shot at doing that. Jonathan had been so excited—the first performance before an audience was in just a few days. How could this be? How could Jonathan not be there? I had no answer.

Jonathan's memorial service took place at the Minetta Lane Theatre. The place was filled to the rafters with sad young faces. Matt found me and asked me to sit with him. He was one of the speakers, and he was very nervous about honoring his friend, about doing him justice. As it was, he was splendid—tender and wise, with wildly funny reminiscences of their shared childhood. Other friends spoke, as did Jonathan's sister, Julie. I have often noticed that memorials are a sad but wonderful way to learn about someone you didn't know very well. I learned a lot about Jonathan Larson that afternoon.

Then the moment came when the cast of the show, those fifteen young people who had sat around me in a circle just a few short days before, got up on the stage. They stood in a straight line from stage left to stage right, looked out at the audience and sang, "Five hundred twenty five thousand six hundred minutes . . . How do you measure a year? . . . How do you measure the life of a man? How about love? Measure in love." Then Adam Pascal, who played Roger—the Rodolfo in this rock version of *La Bohème*—sang, "One song. Glory. One song before I go. One song to leave behind."

My god—Jonathan had written his own memorial!

A few days later I actually saw *Rent* for the first time. I sat next to Matt, who held my hand in a vise that stopped all possible blood flow. Tears were pouring down both our faces. It was all happening up there on the stage. *Jonathan, where are you?!*

Rent is a retelling of *La Bohème*. Instead of taking place in Paris, the setting is New York City's East Village, and instead of the heroine dying of tuberculosis, in Jonathan's version she's dying of AIDS. Part of what made the experience so moving was its immediacy. The characters on the stage were taking the drug AZT, hoping to lengthen their lives, and I'm sure there were people in every audience who were doing exactly the same thing. The score was wonderful, and oh, how those kids could sing!—there were great voices on that stage, and one could just feel that each and every one of them was singing their heart out for Jonathan.

For me there were surprises in the show that quite took my breath away. There was a support group—clearly modeled after the Big Group at Friends In Deed: The phrase "No day but today" was repeated over and over. One night when Jonathan was in the Big Group, a man raised his hand and said that he wasn't really afraid of dying; the thing that bothered him most: Would he lose his dignity? The moment came when one of the actors stepped forward and in the most beautiful voice one could imagine, sang, "Will I lose my dignity?" Then other voices picked up the line until it became a hymn. I assumed Matt was as surprised as I because he seemed equally affected, and, in a very real sense, Friends In Deed belonged to him too. How very elegant of Jonathan not to tell me—to let me discover for myself—those aspects of Friends In Deed that he had included in the show.

I have gone to the theater every chance I've gotten since I was in my teens; I have never seen more powerful audience reactions to a show than that of the *Rent* audiences. There was a very long standing ovation every single night; and opening night on Broadway, as the cast assembled on the stage, there was a standing ovation at the *beginning* of the show. I had certainly never seen that before. Of course the story of Jonathan's shocking death was a strong added element of the experience, but the show was truly inspired and spoke to people in a most powerful way. I wanted everyone in America to see *Rent* and hear what it had to say. *Rent* is about everything we believe in at Friends In Deed. There are gays and straights, there are those who use drugs and those who do not, those who are ill and those who are healthy—and the show does not judge any of it. It is all simply what is. It deals with very tough stuff, and love and compassion are always present.

So much followed that first performance: I saw the show again downtown more than once. I was at the closing night there and at the opening night on Broadway. I took everyone I knew to see it; it wasn't enough to encourage people to go—I wanted to be right there with them. I did a support group with the Boston cast while they were rehearsing in New York; the producers flew me out to California to do a group with the LA cast, to Toronto to do the same thing there. Then, many months later, three of the lead actors went to open the show in London, and again I went with them and facilitated a group with the English cast. I made good friends. I got to know Jonathan's family. I loved every single member of that cast and became close friends with several of them—we, too, have dinners and stay in touch. Anthony Rapp himself came to the Big Group as a client when his mother died, and he is now on Friends In Deed's board of directors.

I have seen *Rent* an embarrassing number of times. One night I saw it with my friend Stephen Sondheim, and afterward as we were walking to dinner, he said, "Did I hear someone say this was your fifteenth time?"

"Fifteen times? Well, that would be crazy, now wouldn't it?"

"Well . . . you couldn't very well tell me . . ."

The whole enormous, involving *Rent* experience showed up at the perfect time in my life. I was still trying hard to find some kind of balance after the loss of Patrick, trying to find out how to be in the world completely on my own. I'd basically gone straight from my father's house to my husband's—this living by myself was a brand-new thing, and while I had great friends and wonderful work and what could definitely be described as a full rich life, it also had some very dark corners. I missed that great crazy Patrick O'Neal. I missed having him to talk to at the end of the day. There was an irresistible pull, every single day, to pick up the phone around 6:00 or 6:30, call him to discuss what we were going to do that evening, and then the daily shock of realizing I couldn't do that.

In the first weeks and months after Patrick died my head was filled with images of illness and hospital rooms. By now those had pretty well faded away, and what I remembered was our life together—mostly the good times. The whole feel and texture of my hours had changed, quieted down a decibel or two. Then along came the exhilaration of *Rent*. Lord knows I had seen other shows multiple times—I'd seen Sondheim shows times beyond counting—but I'd never had that kind of personal involvement before, I'd never been invited to the party in the way that I was with *Rent*—flying to other cities to do groups with the new casts, being in a grief-counseling role around Jonathan's death, falling in love with the extraordinary members of the cast, feeling very much a part of everything that was happening—a big beautiful gift at that so-sad time.

Standing in the crowd after a performance one night, listening to all the excited comments swirling around me, Steve, an FID client, came up to me and said "Well, I think this show should be called *Friends In Deed: The Musical!*"

CHAPTER 19

It was three o'clock in the morning and sleep had abandoned me—flown off into the New York City summer night. I do not like being awake at three o'clock in the morning. It's not my way. I may have trouble falling asleep, but once asleep I stay asleep. Not that night. That night alarm woke me. My first waking thought was, *Am I going to be all right?* Usually I know full well that I am and will be all right. But I didn't know it that night. Not at 3:00 a.m.

My feeling of alarm propelled me out of bed, and there I was standing on a small island of hardwood floor in the middle of a construction site that would one day be my new home. Almost everything I possessed was stacked in the middle of a large square room—a loft in SoHo on the fifth floor of a fine brick building that was built in the mid-1800s—once again, right around the time the Dakota was built (that seems to be my era for New York City homes) to house a factory in what was then the printing district of old New York City. Everywhere I looked there were jagged stacks of lumber, dangling electrical cables that in the half-light could have been snakes hanging from trees, machinery, tools, crushed soda cans left by the workmen, the odd bit of pizza crust, a thick coating of sawdust over all. I was surrounded by shapes and shadows, as if I were in the middle of a Russian Constructivist painting. The huge squares and triangles seemed somewhat sinister, barely illuminated as they were by the lights of the city, the city that wrapped around me outside the great rectangular windows.

It was all strange and unreal. Surreal. How on earth had I come to be here all by myself? How could this be? Patrick and I moved seven times in the years we were married. Seven different times we set up new homes for ourselves and our two sons. Now the boys had their own apartments, and Patrick died almost five years ago.

This would be the first time in my entire long life that I would have a home that was only mine. No one else would live in this loft— only me. I lived alone in my last apartment for four years after Patrick died, but we had moved there together. I could picture him in the various rooms, see him drinking coffee at the table in the kitchen, see him sitting on the leather Chesterfield across from me while we did a recap on the day that was closing, discussed in great detail the film we had just seen. He was there. Well, in truth, I felt his presence in the new space too—I just couldn't really picture him there. But then, I couldn't really picture myself there either.

I think there's a very good chance that I will live alone the rest of my life. For one thing, I'm quite certain that's what I want. I have proven that I can live with; living without seems adventurous and brave—and free. Or that is what I had been thinking and feeling all those last weeks and months of preparing a new home. That night I wasn't quite so sure.

Calling the place a construction site was not an exaggeration. No one in their right mind would have moved into that grimy inhospitable confusion, but having spent many weeks as a house guest in the apartments of three generous friends, I just couldn't do it another minute. Sleeping curled up on a sawdust-covered floor looked more inviting than being somewhere far more comfortable but not my own.

Looking out the north window: Right at my eyeline was a huge advertisement on the side of the building across Houston Street. It covered the entire width of the building and climbed up five stories. It was an ad for Evian water. There was a white footed bathtub just like the one that would be in my new bathroom—should there ever be a new bathroom. In the bathtub sat a very beautiful girl with long brown hair and one perfect leg raised, forming an inverted V, heel resting on the edge of the tub. Around the tub the floor was littered with empty Evian bottles. The beautiful girl looked very happy. I could only assume her happiness was due to her tub being filled with Evian water. The whole ad was white and pale blue and glowed in the night. I found I was comforted by her presence.

Down at the intersection of Houston and Lafayette, there were cars whizzing in every direction—never mind the hour. The whole scene was as New York as New York could be. Charged. Noisy. Was this location a mistake? Had I done the right thing? *Patrick . . . what do you think? Patrick. Talk to me.*

Making a half turn, I looked out the south windows. Across the funny little alley-street below, there's a brick building similar to the one I was standing in. All the windows had beautiful old painted metal shutters that appeared long ago to have been a light blue and were now a time-worn dirty gray. Some were open, some closed, some undecided. I could see into other lofts that had been transformed into apartments; one looked to have a very impressive folk-art collection, which made me curious about the people who lived there, and also, like looking at the Evian girl, the sight of a settled domestic life was somehow reassuring.

Another quarter turn to look out the four huge front windows right into the magnificent Puck Building across Lafayette Street—one of New York's best. Arched windows and below me, over the entranceway, the gilded, chubby little figure of Puck wearing a top hat and a frock coat, outstretched arm holding a hand mirror, gazing at himself. How appropriate to see Puck during that midsummer night's dream—though not really a dream, not dreamy—too much dark nightmare around the edges.

In the past, whenever I envisioned myself as an old woman, living alone, I suddenly became a Brit. I saw myself in a vine-covered English cottage, wearing a classic little cardigan sweater against the chill, reading and writing and drinking endless cups of tea. This image makes no sense whatsoever. I am not drawn to charming little cottages of any nationality, I haven't worn a classic cardigan since high school, and I don't even like tea. So why on earth do I create such a picture? What novel did I once read that put such an idea in my head?

Often, I found myself wanting to say to Patrick, *All right, the joke's over. Come on back now and let's just get on with our life. Just walk in through the door! Alive and well! Enough of this foolishness!* I still have those thoughts.

In those days I sometimes felt as if I were walking along the narrow top of a high wall, concentrating hard on putting one foot carefully in front of the other, arms outstretched for balance. For some reason I remember that night very clearly, and it was one of those times. As I stood and looked around me, what I saw in that room was a kind of visual scream. Usually when I'm having difficulty finding my center, gratitude is the ballast. I reminded myself of my two wonderful sons, of my wealth of extraordinary friends, of the amazing work I am privileged to do. Then I feel better. But not that night.

It was a special joy to be at work during those days because it got me out of the construction zone. I developed a routine. Once I had met the challenge of a sponge bath and dressing, I headed to Balthazar at the corner of Crosby and Spring for morning coffee. It was a good counterbalance. There is nowhere more civilized than Balthazar. At night this gorgeous copy of an upscale French bistro is filled to the rafters with the Prada-clad trendiest of the trendies all shouting at one another above the excruciating din. But in those mornings only a few tables were filled with people quietly reading the paper over their coffee and brioche. Patrick would have loved it. It was beautiful and serene and a good DMZ between the mess I lived in and the intensity of Friends In Deed.

After two café lattes and one fruit focaccia I'd get to my office desk, where there was evidence of my life, past and present, all around me. Dozens and dozens of photographs and notes pinned to the wall in front of me. Photographs of Friends In Deed clients—

many no longer here, many alive and well. Photographs of Patrick and of our sons. Photographs of good friends. Newspaper clippings. Various announcements of dance and theater events. Words of wisdom heard somewhere and hastily written on torn bits of paper. Photographs of the Rent cast. A reproduction of a Sanskrit mandala. A note from my son Max, saying, "Mom, you are so-o-o-o-o-o beautiful!" dropped on my desk just prior to his asking to borrow some money. A note that reads, "Pat O'Neal called to say that he's borrowing a green shirt from you."

I remember that at one point in those living-in-a-construction-site days, the bathtub became the thing—the white cast-iron footed bathtub, like the one in the ad across the street. I thought if I could just get a hot bath, I would look every bit as happy as the girl in the ad, even if my tub was just filled with good old everyday tap water. Patrick would have had a hard time with that situation, too. As opposed to most men, he was a bath taker—showers when there wasn't enough time, but mostly baths—long, long soaks. In the last year of his life, when sleep seemed nearly impossible, there would be baths all night long. I would wake, hear the water running, and, tense with worry, tell myself that if he didn't get more sleep, he would get really ill. Little did I know.

In my eagerness to get out of other people's apartments, I told Fitz that if he could just get me the four walls of a finished painted bedroom with a door that closed, everything else could be managed. When that was accomplished, I huddled in my bedroom—that green island of relative serenity in all the mess. A hundred times a day I would think of something I wanted that was in one of those inaccessible boxes out in the middle of the construction. The furniture had been artfully piled up by the movers, and then, like a city built of blocks in the corner of a first-grade classroom, there were the boxes. Over a hundred book boxes, filled to bursting, nearly fifty china barrels containing all the breakables, two dozen large boxes filled with linens and clothes. My material life. One of the things I kept longing for that I couldn't get my hands on was photographs. I needed to look at photographs of Patrick and our young sons, photographs of the four of us together, photographs of my mother and father and brother. Photographs of myself at other, more glamorous times. Perhaps an instinct for some anchor in this sea on which I seemed to be bobbing up and down—like the proverbial cork in a storm.

At Friends In Deed, we are always encouraging people in the fine art of learning to ask for help, telling us when they're not in good shape. Well, I was not in particularly good shape in those days, and I could see my resistance—I did not want to admit to it. I did not want anyone's help. *Fine! . . . I'm fine! Oh sure, it's a bit tough to live in the middle of construction . . . I guess the August heat does make it more difficult . . . Yes, yes—it is* certainly *a bit weird to be creating a new home without Patrick . . . but I'm fine! I'm really fine!* I could see that I was exactly like all those people at Friends who don't want to ask for help when it's so clear that they need it. I guess it was not so clear that I needed it—everyone seemed to be buying my story.

That September I had a dream about Patrick. It was only the third time since he died that I had dreamed of him. Perhaps there were other times—I'm not good at recalling dreams.

The first two dreams were clear and strong in my memory and they came close together, soon after he died. They were essentially the same dream.

The first took place in a large crowded space that was Friends In Deed–like. Though the look of the place was not the look of the place, it was apparent to me that the people around us were FID clients. The second dream took place in a restaurant where a private party was being held.

In both dreams I was standing in the middle of a lot of people. Patrick walked in, and when I saw him I was startled but not frightened. The people around me began staring at him and whispering to one another. I quickly went to him, feeling the need to explain why people were being so rude—I told him that he was being stared at and whispered about because he had died and so, quite naturally, everyone was a bit shocked to see him.

In both dreams he told me with a slight edge of impatience that he knew perfectly well he had died . . . but as I could see, there he was, standing right in front of me! He seemed to be telling me that his having died had nothing to do with the simple fact that he was there. As I was standing, looking at him, talking to him, touching him— what he was saying seemed unarguably true.

At that time my friends with metaphysical leanings said that quite clearly in these dreams Patrick was visiting me—wanted me to know that he was right here with me, that in truth he hadn't gone anywhere. I am perfectly content with that view of things—it's a profoundly comforting view.

That third dream may well have been prompted in part by the fact that it occurred on Patrick's birthday. In that dream he was there in my new loft on Lafayette Street. He'd just taken a bath and couldn't find his terrycloth robe. I was rather frantically trying to find the box

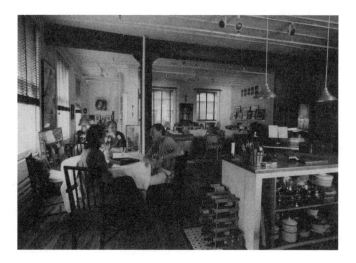

I knew I'd put it in, and I was also trying to hold my tongue about the fact that he was dripping water all over the newly done floor. A down-to-earth dream, nothing fanciful about it, as real as real could be. Perhaps that dream was simply to let me know that he had made this move with me.

CHAPTER 20

The January after Patrick died I joined a weeklong spiritual retreat on the island of St. John. I made the commitment because Ram Dass would be one of the leaders of the retreat, and I figured there was nothing better I could do for my sad broken self than to go to wherever he was.

The minute I stepped off the plane it hit me that I had made the most dreadful mistake I could possibly make. There I was on a hot sweltering Caribbean island, St. John, one of those islands where everyone wants to be—everyone except me. I could not have put myself anywhere that would more painfully show me that I was without Patrick now. I had never been on a tropical island without him before. Not only did it remind me with every hot humid breath I took that Patrick was gone, it also reminded me of all the times he wanted to take an island vacation and I, like a completely selfish bitch, refused to go because tropical islands just aren't really my thing. He would have adored St. John.

We got off the plane, and everything I saw around me was exactly what Patrick would have loved. I stood on the tarmac wondering what on earth I had done, how I could have been so stupid as to think this was a good idea. The lure of Ram Dass had blinded me to the reality of being in the most Patrick of places without Patrick.

My friend Robert was joining the retreat as well, but he was arriving on a later plane. So, when we first landed I was surrounded by dozens of strangers, all of whom were thrilled to be there, all talking to one another, making immediate friends, united in their commitment to the spiritual life. Not me—I was as far off to the side as I could get, hiding behind my very dark glasses, my jaws locked, my entire body in a spasm of grief. I did not want to talk to strangers. I did not want to be friendly. I could barely breathe, let alone say hello or smile.

Soon two very tanned young men appeared to take us to the hotel where the retreat was being held; two large antique yellow buses would carry us to the other side of the island. I found a window seat and immediately began to stare out the window—the most cursory nod to the man who sat down next to me. Sitting there I really didn't quite know how I was going to hold myself together. Seeing Ram Dass would help, but would it help enough? I thought maybe I should get off the bus as fast as I could and simply get on the next plane back to New York. Bit of a shock for Robert when he got there, but he's very resourceful, he'd manage. I kept reminding myself that seeing Ram Dass was certain to be healing, and then in a minute it was too late anyway because the bus had started. I told myself that if I simply couldn't do it I'd get someone to take me back to the airport.

Out the window were all those postcard-island sights: Lush vegetation, little shacks on the side of the road from which the St. John natives watch the happy vacationers come and go, lots of yellow or spotted dogs hanging about the little kids who were staring at our bus while they chewed or drank something with an extremely high sugar content. The bus was bouncing up and down due to a very rutted road and completely inadequate springs. Thick dust everywhere.

The more I looked out the window, the more I saw of tropical island life, the more impossible it was that Patrick was not on that bus with me. I closed my eyes, leaned back, gritted my teeth. *Just get through the next moment. Breathe.*

After about half an hour the bus stopped. At first I thought it was just a normal intersection stop, but then it went on much too long. Now there was a different quality to the talk around me, a rise in pitch, accelerated excitement. I didn't really care enough to look and see what was going on until I heard the driver's heavily accented voice say, "I never see this before . . . I live on this island all my life and I never see this!"

Now I did look. I saw that we were stopped because the ground all around the bus was covered with live iguanas! Dozens of them. Milling about, climbing over one another, completely encircling the bus—great enormous prehistoric lizards. For that moment we were in another age.

Iguanas.

Iguanas.

The Night of the Iguana. *Patrick, are you telling me you are here? Is this your idea of a joke?*

The hotel was not a fancy one. It was built on a hillside that sloped down to the sea, and there was great beauty in all directions. As the hours passed, things did improve. I slowly became a little less demented. Robert arrived—now I had my pal, and that immediately made me feel better. The three-hour sessions with Ram Dass each morning were calming and healing. Just being with him and listening to him reminded me of what I knew in my heart to be true. He reminded me that I was safe, that really everything was all right— Patrick's death, all of it. As Ram Dass said to me right after Patrick died, "There is no such thing as error!" The minute he said it, I knew it was right. Everything was unfolding exactly as was meant, including Patrick's death and my being left on my own. It was all alright. There on that island I began to get back in touch with the truth of that sentence.

Of course Ram Dass, too, reminded me of Patrick—Patrick discovered him in the first place, and ever since he had taken me to that first lecture I had put myself in any room Ram Dass was in whenever that was possible. Now here I was at this impossibly painful time, spending my mornings with Ram Dass and spending my afternoons sitting on an island beach, the last place that, generally speaking, I would ever want to be, watching dozens of people frolic in the brilliant sun and going over in my mind whatever Ram Dass had talked about that morning.

One afternoon, out of the corner of my eye, I saw Ram Dass come onto the beach. I watched as he snaked his way through oiled bodies lying on towels. He made his way to where I was sitting, spread his towel on the sand, and sat down next to me.

We talked of many things as we stared out to sea. We spoke of Patrick and of my life without him; we spoke of AIDS and what there was to learn from this sweeping epidemic; we spoke of Friends In Deed. He asked questions, I asked advice; we spoke of my sons and of his life in California. We even gossiped a bit, about the guru who had disappeared from his New England ashram in a Rolls-Royce with all his devotees' money. As we talked, I was not entirely at ease. I never am in those circumstances. I always feel a bit odd-man-out at spiritual gatherings. For one thing, there is often a lot of name-dropping. Now I have certainly been around world-class name-dropping in Los Angeles and New York, but in these groups, rather than the talk being of dinner with Taylor and Burton, it's all about a month spent on some mountain with Ravi this one or Rimpoche that one, and endless references to great spiritual writings I've not read, all of which make me feel that I'm probably in the wrong place. I did honestly think that Ram Dass thought well of Friends In Deed and the work we do there. But still there was always a bit of feeling like a fraud, even though I recognized in some other participants a bit of pretension around their fine enlightenment. Pretention was not something I'd ever seen in Ram Dass himself. The absolute reverse was true. He never quite seemed to take himself at all seriously.

I guess the weight of feeling that I was probably not the person he thought I was got to me, because I finally said, "You know, I feel as though I need to tell you something. I'm not really a sitter, a meditator. Given your passionate dedication to the practice of meditation, I've always been afraid to tell you that."

"Well, I didn't think you were. You're a dharma yogi. Your work is your practice."

EPILOGUE

In the summer of my eleventh year, we were now living in San Mateo but I went back to the San Fernando Valley for two weeks to stay with my friend Linda, who was also eleven, and who had three brothers and a slender, beautiful divorced mother. They lived in a wonderful old adobe ranch house some blocks from where the Baxter family used to live. Linda's house had all the feel and smell of old California. I dreamed to live in such a house. I thought it exotic to have divorced parents (no one else I knew did). I wished my own mother were thinner.

The highlight of those two weeks was a card game Linda and I played for hours on end. It was called Concentration. We would take a deck of cards, spread them out facedown on the floor and then take turns turning the cards faceup two at a time. The idea was that if I turned over a jack and a jack had been turned over earlier and I could remember where that jack was, I could turn that one over too and the pair would be mine, the goal being to have collected the greater number of pairs at the end of the game. We were obsessed. Barely were our eyes open in the mornings before we had a deck spread out across the floor and were hard at it. I remember that Linda's mother tried to get us to go out into the brilliant summer air—at least for a little while. We could not have been less interested.

Since we resisted stopping the game long enough to take a decent meal break, we often held something edible in one hand while we played—usually something sweet and therefore sticky. Sometimes my hands got so sticky the cards stuck to them, and I remember assigning something vaguely magical to which ones stuck and which did not. I wondered why the nine of clubs stuck to my fingers when

234 | *Talk Softly*

the four of hearts just before had not. Something about that fascinated me.

I'm still fascinated by what sticks in any form. In a long life filled with friends, lovers, foreign cities, restaurants, plates of food, places lived, beloved animals, houses and apartments, wise teachers, beautiful dresses, pretty shoes, gifts given, gifts received, plays and movies, books read, early mornings and late nights—why is it that there are those I can't remember and those I can't forget? What is it about a memory that makes it stick? Logic has nothing to do with it.

There are people I knew for years who are now the dimmest of memories and those I spent a few minutes with long ago who are as vivid as though it were yesterday.

I have cooked meals in many kitchens. For ten years I cooked in my big, fabulously equipped kitchen in the Dakota and I don't recall that experience nearly as well as I do cooking in the second kitchen of my married life: The walls were red enamel, there wasn't much cooking space, and I think I did my very best work there. I made dishes in that tiny space that never turned out so well anywhere else, ever again. Now, why would that be? Why would that be the kitchen that has stuck with me all these years?

When I was about seven years old I went to the house next door and rang the bell. The door was opened by the wife/mother of the house. Her name was Fern. She looked sickly and pale and was wearing a long robe—it was dusty pink and fastened at the waist with four small round buttons of the same color. Now, why the hell would I remember those buttons and know absolutely that there were four of them? Not three, not five—four. Right around that same time I looked out the window one day and saw that same woman's dachshund standing in our yard with one of my beautiful little baby brown rabbits hanging limply from its mouth. I understand full well why I would remember that terrible image, but I can't imagine why the buttons have stuck to my fingers.

In the eighth grade at Park School in San Mateo, we had a teacher named Mrs. Tuttich. She frequently wore a jacket made of crocheted squares in shades of wine red, fuchsia, magenta, and pink. Once, when Patrick was filming a movie in Rome, I sat in an outdoor café in the Piazza Navona every single morning for three months. I sat there drinking cappuccino and watching the life in the piazza. My memory of the buildings and the fountains is extremely cloudy, almost no specific detail—I remember every stitch of Mrs. Tuttich's jacket. I carry the image of that jacket with me everywhere I go. I would so much rather carry the Piazza Navona. Again—why?

It can be such a tiny moment that makes all the difference. When I was four years old my mother took me on the train east to Ohio, first to Lorain, to the Hungarian community where she'd grown up so that I could meet her parents, and then to Toledo, where her half-sister lived with her husband, Gary. One evening we must have gone out to dinner, and now we were headed back to their house. Gary was carrying me on his shoulders. It was dark and it had rained, so that from my high perch I could see the shine of rain on the streets and the cars illuminated by tall golden streetlights. What I saw and felt had nothing to do with anything I knew back home—streets of California ranch-house suburbs lit only by the stars at night—a feeling of emptiness. These houses were close together, and there was the sense of a lot of people nearby, things were happening around me. It was exciting and glamorous and I knew in my little four-year-old heart that it was everything I wanted—glittery and mysterious. Now every single time I am out at night on a New York City street after a rainfall, that moment on Uncle Gary's shoulders comes flooding back. I often think it's the most powerful memory I have— it almost feels like a blow—it was such a very small moment.

But, here's what I know: Every single experience that I have ever had—whether I remember it or not—is a part of where and who I am right this minute.

I have a tattoo of a beautiful bird on my left shoulder. I come to have a tattoo because my wonderful brother happens to be one of the world's greatest living experts on the art of the tattoo, his sons are tattoo artists, and it seemed like the "family" thing to do. The facts notwithstanding, it is completely improbable that coming from where I started, I would ever have a tattoo. It is equally improbable that I would, on a weekly basis, stand in front of a large roomful of people dealing with life-threatening illness and/or heartbreak. The fact that that's what I do is beyond logic and makes perfect sense in equal measure. I know absolutely that these things are the result of every single thing that has ever happened to me in my long life—all of it is a part of the answer to Patrick's question: "When did this happen?" Whether it appears to stick or not—every bit of it matters.

ACKNOWLEDGMENTS

THANK YOU

There would be no book if Patrick hadn't asked me—When did this happen? For that and so much more . . .

I will always be grateful to Archie and Drew for including me in that extraordinary time.

Along the way, there were friends who read pages or chapters and gave me valuable feedback. That list must certainly include Robert, Mark, James, Cybele, Brendan, Danielle, Jordan, Kate, Anthony, and, of course, Mike. I particularly thank brilliant Christopher for all his time and care.

Bill is the best agent in the whole world—it's as simple as that. And he always wants to go to the movies.

Seven Stories Press felt like home the minute I walked in. It is an honor and a pleasure to work with Dan. Also with Veronica, Ruth, and all the other wonderful people down there on Watts Street.

It amazes me that Linda and Michael consistently ask me about my book—how can it be that they are asking *me* about *my* book? It doesn't make any sense.

The same could be said of Alice and Michael.

The staff of Friends In Deed is the best staff there could ever be and have supported me every inch of the way: Robert, Cynthia, Read, Eric, Michelle, and Michael. From my heart, thank you.

I thank John for the miraculous studio where he painted and I wrote—hours I will never forget.

There are also those dear friends who have never read a word, but have talked to me about this project and are always on my side, which makes all the difference. That list would start with my wonderful brother, Rob, and continue with Phyllis, John, Joel, Jean, Victor, Christina, John, Peter, Hebe, Steve, James, Paul, Danny, Raul, Sam, Chris, and Mike, and those I can't remember at this moment but will the minute this book has gone to press and it's too late.

I must thank my two adored sons, Max and Fitz, who keep my life a noisy one, which I suspect is good for me.

And how could I not acknowledge the three glorious animals who live with me—or, more accurately, on top of me: Bird, Blue, and Louie?

I thank each and every client who has ever walked through the door of Friends In Deed—my teachers, all.

PHOTOGRAPHY CREDITS AND PERMISSIONS

Page 9: The O'Neal family. Photograph by Bill King.

Page 22: Fig, the cat; Moon, the dog; and me. Photograph by Patrick O'Neal.

Page 32: Archie and Drew. Photograph by Cordelia Anderson.

Page 67: Patrick, when I met him. Photograph by Clifford Coffin.

Page 69: Modeling. Photograph by Claude Virgin.

Page 73: The California kid. Photograph by Robert Earl Baxter.

Page 74: Robert Earl Baxter, Helen Komaromy Baxter. Photographs courtesy of Cynthia O'Neal.

Page 98: Michael with China and Bosco. Photograph courtesy of the Freiberg family.

Page 105: Cast of *The Ginger Man*: Marian Seldes, Stefan Gierasch, Patrick O'Neal, Margaret Phillips. Photograph by Tom Palumbo. Courtesy of the Patricia Bosworth Collection.

Page 108: The original Ginger Man. Photograph courtesy of Cynthia O'Neal.

Page 121: The Dakota. Photograph courtesy of Cynthia O'Neal.

Page 124: Phyllis and Patrick, Lenny and me. Photographs courtesy of Phyllis Newman.

Page 151: Ram Dass. Photograph courtesy of Cynthia O'Neal.

Page 169: The three sisters: Donaly, Pamela, and Victoria. Photograph by Carolyn Jones.

Page 177: My Hungarian mother. Photograph courtesy of Cynthia O'Neal.

Page 180: Backstage with Nureyev—the first time. Photograph by V. Sladon.

Page 228: My loft. Photograph by Clovis França.

ABOUT THE AUTHOR

Cynthia O'Neal is the founder and president of Friends In Deed, a New York City crisis center that provides emotional and spiritual support for anyone diagnosed with HIV/AIDS, cancer, and other life-threatening illnesses. This is her first book.